The Doctor, the Engineer, and the AI:
How We Created a Breakthrough Technology to Beat Cancer

LYFBLEND LLC

LYFBLEND LLC

601 Cleveland Str, Suite 310, Clearwater, Florida 33755, USA

https://lyfblend.com/

ISBN: 979-8-218-50187-7

To April and Isabell,

Your unwavering love, strength, and support have been the pillars that sustained us on this journey. As we delved into thousands of pages of research, debated long into the night, and sought to bridge the worlds of medicine, technology, and hope, your belief in our mission never wavered.

This book is more than a testament to scientific progress and AI-driven innovation in cancer care—it is a reflection of the patience, dedication, and compassion you have so generously given. Without your encouragement, understanding, and tireless support, none of this would have been possible.

With deepest love and gratitude,
Dean Silver, MD, MD (H) & Andreas Kazmierczak, MS

Publisher: LYFBLEND LLC, Florida USA

ISBN 979-8-218-50187-7

Title: The Doctor, the Engineer, and the AI -
How We Created a Breakthrough Technology to Beat Cancer

Frist Edition: March 2025
Printed in the United States of America

Authors:
Dr Dean Silver, MD, MD (H), Andreas Kazmierczak, MS

Disclaimer:

The information in this book is for informational purposes only and should not be considered as professional medical advice. Always consult with a qualified healthcare professional before starting any new treatment.

This book is a work of fiction inspired by real-world ideas and advancements. While the characters of Dr. Dean and Andreas share names with the authors, they are not direct representations of any real individuals. Many details, events, and personalities have been altered, fictionalized, or combined to create a compelling narrative.

Any resemblance to actual persons, living or deceased, is purely coincidental. The book introduces other characters who may seem similar to real people, but they, too, are fictionalized for storytelling purposes. This is not a factual account but rather an exploration of possibilities in the fight against cancer.

Contents

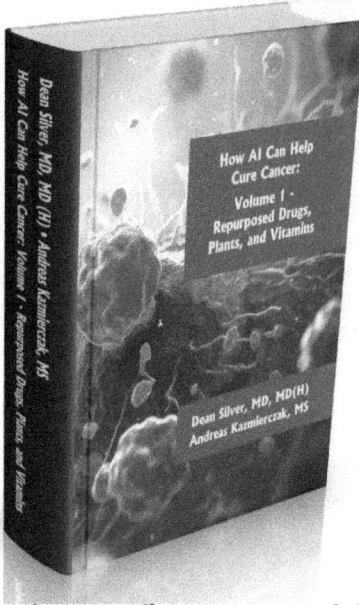

Book recommendation:

How AI Can Help Cure Cancer: Volume 1 - Repurposed Drugs, Plants, and Vitamins
Dean Silver MD, MD (H)   Andreas Kazmierczak, MS

ISBN Paperback   979-8-9916163-0-0
ISBN EPUB   979-8-9916163-1-7

In "How AI Can Help Cure Cancer: Volume 1 - Repurposed Drugs, Plants, and Vitamins", Dean Silver MD, MD(H) and AI scientist Andreas Kazmierczak MS explore the groundbreaking role of artificial intelligence in integrative cancer treatment. This book reveals how AI-driven analysis is revolutionizing cancer care by identifying the most effective repurposed drugs, plant-based therapies, and vitamins to combat the disease.

Dr. Silver, a leading integrative oncologist, shares his personal journey of overcoming cancer and staying in remission for 25 years using innovative, non-toxic therapies. Kazmierczak, an expert in AI, has trained the CANCERASE AI on over 300,000 pages (as of February 2025) of medical data, offering a powerful tool for personalized cancer treatment. Together, they present a cutting-edge approach that moves beyond conventional high-dose chemotherapy, reducing harmful side effects while improving outcomes. With rapid advancements in AI and major investments in medical technology, this book provides hope and practical guidance for those seeking smarter, more effective cancer treatments.

This book represents a new genre in medical literature—an AI-validated, evidence-based compendium of cancer research. Unlike conventional medical texts, it merges the power of artificial intelligence with extensive scientific validation to create a dynamic, up-to-date resource for cancer treatment. It is neither purely academic nor solely practical; instead, it bridges the gap between cutting-edge research and clinical application, providing a definitive, data-driven approach to oncology.

This book is a groundbreaking reference in the field of cancer treatment, providing an unbiased, scientifically validated overview of the latest advancements in oncology. Unlike traditional books, this work is entirely grounded in scientific evidence, ensuring that every statement and recommendation is backed by rigorous research. The content is verified using our proprietary medical AI (CANCERASE GPT, visit cangpt.ai), which has been trained on over 300,000 pages of research proceedings and scientific materials.

A must-read for patients, caregivers, and medical professionals looking to harness AI in the fight against cancer.

Author Dean Silver MD, MD (H)

Dr. Dean Silver is a distinguished physician with over 48 years of experience in hospital-based medicine. Initially trained as a traditional cardiologist, he later expanded his expertise to include integrative and precision medicine, blending conventional and alternative therapies to enhance health and extend patient lifespans.

His medical journey took a transformative turn 25 years ago when he was diagnosed with lymphoma—likely a result of excessive radiation exposure in the cardiac cath lab, chronic stress, sleep deprivation, and an unhealthy diet. Refusing to rely solely on conventional treatments, he embarked on a global search for advanced integrative oncology approaches. Through a combination of targeted, metabolic-based therapies, he successfully overcame cancer and remains cancer-free to this day.

Dr. Silver earned his medical degree from Temple University School of Medicine, followed by a three-year internal medicine residency at Albert Einstein Medical Center. He then completed a fellowship in invasive cardiology, establishing himself as a respected cardiologist before shifting his focus to cancer treatment.

For the past 25 years, Dr. Silver has dedicated his career to integrative oncology, pioneering breakthrough therapies for stage IV cancers, metastases, and treatment-resistant tumors. His innovative approach treats cancer as a metabolic disease, targeting its root causes rather than just its symptoms.

His cutting-edge protocols incorporate:

- Hyperbaric oxygen therapy

- Hyperthermia

- Cryoablation

- Metronomic low-dose chemotherapy

- Chemo-sensitivity testing

- PEMF (Pulsed Electromagnetic Field Therapy)

- And other advanced treatments

These strategies have led to remarkable remissions in patients with stage IV cancer, offering new hope where traditional treatments have failed.

Dr. Silver is also at the forefront of integrative oncology research, playing a key role in the development of CANCERASE AI, the world's first AI-driven cancer treatment system. His work focuses on collecting and analyzing medical data to enhance AI-driven cancer diagnostics and treatment protocols, with the ultimate goal of revolutionizing global cancer care.

Outside of medicine, Dr. Silver is passionate about golf and tennis. He and his fiancée are actively involved in charitable initiatives, supporting humanitarian and health-focused causes in Florida, where they reside.

Author Andreas Kazmierczak, MS

M.Sc. Eng. Andreas Kazmierczak is the founder of Expert Robotics LLC and BackToCAD AI Technologies LLC, two U.S.-based companies specializing in AI software development. He also serves as a director on the board of the IntelliCAD Technology Consortium. With a career in software development spanning over four decades, Andreas has built extensive expertise through his university education, postgraduate training, and hands-on experience in AI, robotics, and CAD technology.

Andreas earned his Master's Degree in Engineering from the prestigious Technical University in Aachen, Germany, where he developed a strong foundation in numerical mathematics and efficient programming techniques. During his studies, he worked as a scientific assistant in the Department of Hydrology and Statistics, successfully developing AI expert systems for hydrology. Later, he delivered lectures and training sessions on artificial intelligence and statistical methods at the university.

For over 35 years, Andreas has been a pioneer in CAD software development through his German company, Kazmierczak Software GmbH, which has provided innovative solutions for the CAD industry. His software is widely used worldwide, with over 100,000 paid users and more than one million unpaid users. He also holds numerous patents in data security and data exchange methods. As a recognized industry expert, he is a member of the Association of Consulting Engineers (VBI), Germany's leading professional organization for independent consulting and planning engineers.

Andreas is also a prolific author, having written over eight books in both German and English on computer-aided design (CAD) and artificial intelligence systems. His books have been widely used by engineers, AI researchers, and technology professionals.

Currently, Andreas resides in Florida, USA, where he is an active supporter of various charity organizations, dedicated to helping those in need and contributing to community-driven initiatives.

His interest in AI-driven cancer treatment was sparked by a personal case and connections with leading medical professionals working in integrative oncology. This profound experience led him to develop CANCERASE AI, an advanced artificial intelligence system designed to revolutionize cancer treatment by combining the most sophisticated medical knowledge with groundbreaking AI technology.

CANCERASE AI has rapidly gained worldwide recognition, attracting support from private individuals, the medical sector, industry leaders, and government organizations. The project is expanding into a global cancer treatment initiative with the potential to heal thousands—if not millions—of people within the next 5 to 10 years. As the project continues to grow at an unprecedented pace, this AI-driven breakthrough is poised to reshape the future of cancer care worldwide.

In addition to his groundbreaking work in AI and software development, Andreas is a talented classical pianist, specializing in the works of Chopin, Beethoven, and Debussy. He regularly performs concerts in Germany and the United States and shares his music through widely viewed online performances.

Andreas is also a devoted husband and father of four children, balancing his passion for technology, music, and humanitarian efforts with family life.

Introduction

"The greatest breakthroughs begin where the impossible meets the unthinkable. To truly defeat cancer, we must challenge everything we know, break free from outdated dogma, and embrace a future where knowledge, technology, and human resilience converge. The answers have always been there—hidden in plain sight. This book will unveil them." Andreas Kazmierczak

This is not just another book about cancer. It is a revelation—one that will forever change the way you perceive this disease. What if everything you've been told about cancer treatment was only a fraction of the truth? What if the cure has been hidden in the shadows, waiting for the right moment to emerge?

For years, cancer has been seen as an unbeatable force, a relentless enemy that can only be subdued through toxic, often brutal methods. But what if we told you that the war against cancer has been fought on the wrong battlefield? That beyond chemotherapy, radiation, and surgery lies a deeper truth—one that science, technology, and ancient wisdom are now uncovering?

This book is the product of two minds from opposite worlds—a traditionally trained physician and an AI engineer—who found themselves standing on the same precipice, facing the same enemy: cancer. One of us lived in the rigid structure of conventional medicine, armed with decades of clinical experience. The other thrived in the fast-paced evolution of artificial intelligence, where limitless data reveals hidden patterns and exposes suppressed truths. Separately, we followed the paths dictated by our professions. But cancer changed everything.

When we became patients ourselves, we realized that the conventional treatments we once trusted held only part of the answer. We saw firsthand how the system operates—how it clings to outdated protocols, dismisses promising discoveries, and resists change. We learned that cancer is not just a disease of the body—it is a biological puzzle, a complex and intelligent force that requires an equally sophisticated response.

So we asked the unthinkable: What if we combined the power of AI with the deepest knowledge of integrative medicine? Could we uncover a new path—one that doesn't just treat cancer but deciphers its very nature, exposing its vulnerabilities and dismantling its power?

The answer was more astonishing than we had ever imagined.

A New Era of Cancer Treatment

Through our research, we discovered something extraordinary—something that challenges the very foundation of cancer treatment. Hidden within thousands of studies, buried in forgotten research papers, and scattered across the wisdom of ancient healing traditions, we found a pattern. A convergence of knowledge that, when pieced together with the precision of AI, forms a revolutionary new paradigm.

We are at the dawn of a medical revolution. AI is no longer just a tool for technology—it is the key to unlocking the deepest mysteries of cancer. With its ability to analyze vast amounts of data, AI can identify hidden correlations, detect weaknesses in cancer's defenses, and design personalized treatment strategies in ways no human mind could achieve alone.

This book will take you on a journey unlike any other. It will challenge your understanding of cancer, unveil suppressed discoveries, and introduce you to the future of medicine—where AI-driven intelligence works alongside doctors and patients to create highly individualized treatment plans. It will reveal therapies that have been overlooked, dismissed, or hidden from public knowledge, yet hold the potential to transform lives.

A Guide for the Seekers of Truth

If you or a loved one has been touched by cancer, you have likely heard the words *"There's nothing more we can do."* But what if that wasn't true? What if the answer has been waiting all along—simply ignored or dismissed because it doesn't fit within the conventional model of care?

This book is for those who refuse to accept limitations. For the patients seeking real answers, for the doctors willing to look beyond their textbooks, and for the skeptics who need proof before they believe. It is for those who sense, deep down, that something has been missing from the conversation about cancer for far too long.

Here, you will find more than just theories—you will find solutions. We will take you inside the revolutionary research that is rewriting everything we know about cancer. You will discover groundbreaking insights into:

- The hidden biological nature of cancer and why conventional medicine has misunderstood it.
- How AI is uncovering patterns in cancer that human doctors could never detect.
- The suppressed role of repurposed drugs that have been quietly shown to fight cancer but never entered mainstream treatment.
- How metabolic therapies, immune system activation, and

personalized nutrition can be the missing pieces in your cancer-fighting arsenal.

- The global advancements in cancer treatment that are years ahead of standard protocols in the West.

This is not just another cancer book. This is the book that will change how you see cancer forever.

The Future is Here—And You Are Part of It

We are standing on the edge of something extraordinary. The knowledge contained in these pages is not speculation—it is real, tested, and ready to be used. But knowledge alone is not enough. The true power lies in what you do with it.

Together, we can break the cycle of outdated treatments and usher in a new era of healing. Together, we can expose the gaps in conventional care and replace them with precision-driven, AI-enhanced strategies. Together, we can change the way cancer is treated—not years from now, but today.

This is not just our journey. It is yours. The answers are here. The choice is yours. Are you ready to see what has been hidden from you all along?

Welcome to the future of cancer treatment.

Further Reading: A Must-Read After This Book

In this book, we have introduced the revolutionary concept of using AI-driven integrative medicine to fight cancer. We have explored how CANCERASE AI is paving the way for a new era in oncology—one that moves beyond conventional treatments and incorporates the best of modern science, personalized medicine, and holistic approaches.

But as groundbreaking as this vision is, there is so much more to learn. Cancer is a complex, multi-faceted disease, and its treatment requires a deep understanding of every possible tool at our disposal—from cutting-edge pharmaceuticals to the healing power of nature.

For those who are ready to dive deeper into the science of integrative oncology, we highly recommend our comprehensive 500-page guide:

"How AI Can Help Cure Cancer: Volume 1 - Repurposed Drugs, Plants, and Vitamins"
Dr. Dean Silver, MD, MD (H) & Andreas Kazmierczak , MS

This monumental work serves as an encyclopedia of integrative cancer treatments, detailing every known repurposed drug, plant-based therapy, and essential vitamin that has shown promise in fighting cancer. Whether you are a patient, a caregiver, a medical professional, or a researcher, this book provides a treasure trove of knowledge—all backed by scientific research, clinical studies, and real-world success stories.

What You Will Discover in This Book:

Repurposed Drugs: Learn how existing medications—originally developed for other diseases—are being successfully used to starve tumors, block metastasis, and enhance traditional treatments. From metformin and statins to anti-parasitic drugs and low-dose chemotherapy, you will find an in-depth analysis of their cancer-fighting potential.

The Power of Medicinal Plants: Nature has always provided potent anti-cancer compounds. This book delves into thousands of plants and their extracts, including:

- Curcumin from turmeric—one of the most powerful natural anti-inflammatory agents.

- Artemisinin—a compound from sweet wormwood that selectively kills cancer cells.

- Berberine—a plant alkaloid that works similarly to metformin, reducing cancer cell growth.

- Resveratrol, Quercetin, and EGCG—polyphenols with strong anti-cancer effects.

Vitamins and Minerals in Cancer Therapy: Discover how high-dose vitamin C, vitamin D, selenium, zinc, and magnesium can play a role in enhancing immunity, reducing inflammation, and making cancer cells more vulnerable to treatment.

Why This Book is Essential

Cancer patients and doctors alike are beginning to recognize the power of integrative medicine. Traditional treatments like chemotherapy and radiation often fail to address the root causes of cancer, leaving patients vulnerable to recurrence. This book explores the science behind a metabolic and holistic approach, showing how combining repurposed drugs, plant-based medicine, and essential nutrients can maximize survival and quality of life.

With over 500 pages of meticulously researched information, this book is designed to be the ultimate resource for anyone serious about understanding every available tool in the fight against cancer.

Our work with CANCERASE AI is just the beginning. Artificial intelligence is revolutionizing medicine, and books like "How AI Can Help Cure Cancer: Volume 1" are paving the way for evidence-based, data-driven treatments that integrate the best of modern and natural medicine.

If you are looking for a comprehensive guide that will help you or your loved ones understand and implement integrative cancer therapies, this book is an essential read. It provides actionable knowledge that can be applied immediately— whether you're working with an oncologist or exploring alternative therapies.

Where to Get This Book

"How AI Can Help Cure Cancer: Volume 1 - Repurposed Drugs, Plants, and Vitamins" is available as a print edition and digital format. You can find it through major bookstores, medical publishers, amazon.com, lulu.com, and online retailers.

Knowledge is power—and when it comes to cancer, having the right information can mean the difference between life and death. We invite you to explore this groundbreaking resource and take control of your health with the most advanced, science-based integrative treatments available today.

Chapter 1: A Chance Meeting in the IV Room - How Cancerase GPT Was Born

"Sometimes, the most groundbreaking ideas are born in the most unexpected places. Adversity is not an end—it is the spark that ignites innovation, turning struggle into purpose and knowledge into hope." Andreas Kazmierczak

Dr. Dean had spent decades in hospitals and clinics, treating patients with heart problems and, later, with cancer. He knew the sterile scent of antiseptic too well, and the constant beeping of machines was the soundtrack to his life. But there he was, sitting in an IV room, not as a doctor but as a patient receiving alternative integrative cancer care. Life has a funny way of turning the tables.

Meanwhile, across the room, Andreas, a sharp-minded AI engineer, was staring at his own IV drip. He wasn't used to being still—his mind was usually racing at a thousand miles an hour, filled with algorithms and data points. But cancer had a way of forcing even the busiest minds to slow down.

He had been diagnosed with a type of cancer that, at first, he didn't think was a big deal. "I'm healthy," he thought, "I eat well, I work hard. Cancer doesn't happen to people like me." But here he was, learning the hard way that cancer doesn't discriminate.

The two men sat in silence, each lost in their thoughts. Dr. Dean was mentally organizing his knowledge about integrative cancer treatments, wondering how he could share what he had learned over the years with more people. Andreas was contemplating his own journey, realizing that his cancer was finally going into remission after trying several integrative therapies, including this IV treatment that seemed to take forever.

As an engineer, Andreas found the lengthy treatment sessions frustratingly slow and inefficient. "There has to be a faster way to learn about all these different treatments," he thought, watching the drip, drip, drip of the IV.

It was during one of these long sessions that Andreas noticed Dr. Dean across the room, shuffling through a thick stack of papers. Curiosity got the better of him. "Hey, looks like you've got enough papers there to write a book," Andreas joked, trying to break the ice.

Dr. Dean chuckled. "Well, funny you say that. I've been thinking about doing just that—organizing all this knowledge and experience I've gathered over the years. But there's just so much. It feels like an impossible task."

Andreas nodded, "I know the feeling. I've been through dozens of treatments, some conventional, some very unconventional. And now that I'm finally in remission, I'm wondering how I can share what I've learned with others, to help them navigate this journey more easily."

There was a pause as the two men considered each other's words. Then Andreas's eyes lit up. "Wait a minute," he said, a spark of excitement in his voice. "I've got an idea. You know, I work with AI—artificial intelligence. What if we created an AI that could answer any question about integrative cancer care? It could combine all your knowledge and experience with data from all over the world. We could help people find the information they need quickly, without having to go through stacks of papers or endless research."

Dr. Dean raised an eyebrow. "An AI for cancer care? How would that even work?"

Andreas leaned forward, now fully animated. "It's like this: imagine a machine that's constantly learning, just like a human, but it never sleeps and never forgets. It could analyze data from thousands of studies, integrate different treatment methods, and provide personalized suggestions based on a person's unique situation. We could feed it all the information you have—your experience, your research, everything—and it would keep learning and adapting as new treatments come out."

Dr. Dean smiled, intrigued by the idea. "That sounds... revolutionary. But can it really be done?"

Andreas grinned. "Why not? I've got time," he said, pointing to the IV drip. "And honestly, these treatments give me plenty of time to think. Why not put that time to good use?"

Over the next few weeks, the two men began to collaborate. During their long IV sessions, they brainstormed, shared stories, and pieced together a vision for what would become Cancerase GPT, the world's first AI dedicated entirely to integrative cancer care.

Andreas, with his laptop balanced on his knees and IV drip by his side, started coding the framework for the AI. Meanwhile, Dr. Dean began feeding the AI with all his accumulated knowledge, research, and experience, from the latest studies in nutritional science to ancient healing practices.

They worked tirelessly, and despite the seriousness of their situation, they found ways to keep things light. "If this AI thing doesn't work out, we can always open a clinic called 'Dr. Dean and the Machine,'" Andreas joked one day, earning a hearty laugh from Dr. Dean. They became an odd couple, united by their shared experience with cancer and a newfound mission to change how people access cancer treatment information.

Finally, after months of hard work, Cancerase GPT was born. It wasn't just a tool—it was a revolutionary step forward in cancer care. Now, anyone, anywhere in the world, could ask Cancerase GPT about integrative cancer treatments, and it would provide answers based on the latest scientific research and centuries-old wisdom.

As word of Cancerase GPT spread, it quickly became clear that they had created something special. Patients, doctors, and caregivers alike began using it to explore new treatment options, find nutritional advice, and learn about therapies they had never considered. For the first time, there was a tool that combined the best of human knowledge with the endless learning capabilities of AI.

Andreas and Dr. Dean knew they were just scratching the surface of what AI could do for cancer care. "We've opened the door," Dr. Dean said one day, looking at the growing database of Cancerase GPT. "Now it's up to the world to walk through it."

And walk through it they did. The AI continued to grow, learning from each query and constantly updating itself with the latest research. For patients, it was a source of hope and empowerment. For doctors, it was a tool that provided new methods and possibilities. And for Andreas and Dr. Dean, it was proof that even in the darkest times, there is always a chance for innovation, collaboration, and a brighter future.

Their journey from an IV room to creating a groundbreaking AI was a testament to the power of resilience, creativity, and the belief that sometimes, the best ideas come from the most unexpected places. And so, Cancerase GPT became a beacon of hope, not just for those battling cancer today, but for all those who would face the disease in the future.

In the end, Andreas looked back on his time in the IV room with a smile. "Who would've thought," he mused, "that a slow IV drip would lead to something that might one day help cure cancer?" Dr. Dean laughed, "Sometimes, the slowest roads lead to the most incredible destinations."

And with that, they continued their work, driven by the knowledge that they were part of something much bigger than themselves—a revolution in the way the world thinks about, fights, and ultimately, beats cancer.

Chapter 2: Coding in the IV Room - The Birth of Cancerase GPT

"Great innovations are born not in perfect conditions, but in moments of struggle, necessity, and determination. When knowledge meets purpose, even an IV room can become the birthplace of a revolution." Andreas Kazmierczak

The soft hum of medical machines and the occasional beep from a monitor filled the IV room. Andreas, the AI engineer, was nestled in his chair with a laptop balanced precariously on his knees. The IV drip attached to his arm was delivering a cocktail of integrative therapies designed to help his body fight cancer. Four hours a day, he sat there, not just as a patient but as a coder on a mission. His fingers danced across the keyboard, writing lines of Python code and piecing together a revolutionary AI he named Cancerase GPT.

Across the room, Dr. Dean was hunched over a stack of papers, scribbling furiously. He was determined to compile every bit of knowledge he had gathered over decades about integrative cancer treatments. "This might be the only way to get all this information in one place," he thought, glancing over at Andreas. "And if anyone can do it, it's him."

Andreas was deep into coding with LangChain, a framework that allowed him to build powerful AI models. He was setting up connections, creating neural networks, and using natural language processing—all while getting his daily dose of IV treatment. Every day, Andreas would code for hours, then meet with Dr. Dean to discuss the latest findings and how they could be integrated into the AI. It was an unlikely partnership, forged in a shared battle against cancer and a desire to make a difference.

"What's Pinecone?" Dr. Dean asked one day, noticing Andreas's screen filled with lines of code and a name he didn't recognize.

"It's a vector database," Andreas explained, not taking his eyes off his laptop. "We're going to use it to store all this knowledge you've been gathering. By vectorizing the data—essentially turning it into mathematical representations—we can make sure Cancerase GPT can understand and recall this information efficiently. Think of it like teaching the AI to have a photographic memory, but with your medical knowledge and all these scientific articles."

Dr. Dean nodded, still a bit mystified by the tech jargon but excited about the possibilities. "And once it's in there, it can learn from it all? Even the stuff we're adding now?"

"Exactly," Andreas said, his fingers still flying over the keyboard. "We're training Cancerase GPT on massive datasets, thousands of internet pages, and hundreds of scientific articles. Once it's done, it'll know almost everything humans have discovered about integrative cancer treatment. And the best part? It'll be able to analyze this information to find new treatment methods, create nutritional blends tailored to cancer care, and help plan better treatment strategies using vitamins, nutrition, and other integrative approaches."

Day by day, Andreas coded through his treatments, the IV drip serving as a constant reminder of why this project was so important. He built models and tweaked algorithms, all while his body was receiving treatments that he hoped would keep his cancer in remission. His laptop became a symbol of hope, not just for himself but for every cancer patient searching for answers.

Dr. Dean continued to compile his decades of experience,

filling notebooks with insights and data. "Here's something interesting," he said one day, holding up a page. "A study from Japan on the use of specific herbs in conjunction with chemotherapy. The results were quite promising."

Andreas nodded, "Perfect. I'll make sure Cancerase GPT can integrate that into its recommendations. It's exactly the kind of synergy we want to capture—combining the best of traditional and modern medicine."

After months of relentless work and collaboration, Cancerase GPT was finally ready. Andreas and Dr. Dean had trained the AI on an incredible amount of data, making it one of the most knowledgeable resources on integrative cancer treatment ever created. It could answer questions, suggest treatment options, recommend nutritional plans, and even propose new blends of vitamins and supplements tailored to specific types of cancer.

But Andreas and Dr. Dean weren't satisfied with keeping this tool to themselves. "We need to share this," Andreas said one day, looking up from his laptop with a determined expression. "We've got something incredible here, something that could change how the world treats cancer. We have to give it away, make it available to everyone—doctors, patients, families."

Dr. Dean smiled, a sense of pride swelling in his chest. "I agree. This knowledge shouldn't be hidden away. It should be a gift to mankind—a free tool that anyone can use to fight cancer more effectively."

And so, Cancerase GPT was released as a free resource to the world. They built a simple, user-friendly website where anyone could ask the AI questions about integrative cancer treatments and get tailored advice. Whether it was a doctor looking for the latest research on herbal therapies or a patient trying to find the best nutritional plan during chemotherapy, Cancerase GPT was there, ready to help.

The response was overwhelming. Stories began pouring in from all over the globe—patients who had found new hope, doctors who had discovered new methods, and families who felt empowered with knowledge. Cancerase GPT became more than just an AI; it became a symbol of hope and collaboration in the fight against cancer.

"We did it," Andreas said one day, as he and Dr. Dean sat in their usual spots in the IV room. "We actually did it."

Dr. Dean nodded, looking around at the familiar room where it all began. "Yeah, we did. And this is just the beginning. We've started something here that will outlive us, something that will keep learning and evolving."

Andreas grinned, "Who knew a laptop and an IV drip could lead to this?"

They both laughed, their spirits lifted by the thought. It had been a long journey, filled with challenges and uncertainty, but they had created something that would make a difference. Cancerase GPT was not just a tool but a revolution—a testament to what can happen when science, technology, and human determination come together.

And in giving Cancerase GPT to the world, they gave something far more valuable than just an AI. They gave hope, a new way forward, and the promise of a future where cancer could be met with knowledge, courage, and endless possibility.

As the world embraced Cancerase GPT, Andreas and Dr. Dean knew that this was only the beginning. The AI would continue to learn, adapt, and grow, just like the patients it was designed to help. And in doing so, it would forever change the landscape of cancer treatment.

And with that, they settled back in their chairs, ready for whatever came next, confident that they had made a lasting impact on the world. And all it took was a laptop, a drip, and a whole lot of determination.

Chapter 3: Unpacking the Power of AI - How Andreas Explained AI to Dr. Dean

"True progress is born at the intersection of knowledge and curiosity. When medicine and technology unite, we unlock new possibilities—not just for answers, but for a future where healing knows no boundaries." Andreas Kazmierczak

In the IV room, amid the gentle hum of machines and the rhythmic drip of IVs, Andreas and Dr. Dean continued their work. Dr. Dean, though a seasoned physician, was new to the world of artificial intelligence. He had been curious about how their AI, Cancerase GPT, was actually built. Andreas, ever patient and eager to share, decided to break it down for him in the simplest terms possible.

"Alright, Dr. Dean," Andreas began, setting his laptop aside for a moment, "let's start with the basics of AI. AI, or artificial intelligence, is a way to make computers think and learn like humans. It's about teaching machines to understand patterns and data, so they can make decisions or predictions."

Dr. Dean nodded, his brows furrowing in concentration. "I get the general idea, but how does this apply to what we're doing with Cancerase GPT?"

Andreas leaned back, taking a deep breath. "Great question. What we're doing is using a type of AI called a Large Language Model, or LLM. An LLM, like ChatGPT-4, is designed to understand and generate human language. It's been trained on vast amounts of text from the internet, books, articles—pretty much anything you can think of. This training allows it to understand context, answer questions, and even generate text like it's having a conversation with you."

Dr. Dean raised an eyebrow. "So, ChatGPT-4 is just... a very smart program that can chat like a human?"

"Exactly," Andreas said, smiling. "But it's more than just chatting. It's understanding the nuances of language, learning from every interaction, and generating responses that are contextually relevant. It's like having a conversation with someone who's read almost every book and article ever written. And the 4.0 version we're using is even more advanced—it's better at understanding complex questions and providing detailed, accurate responses."

Dr. Dean was intrigued. "That's impressive. But how do we make sure Cancerase GPT knows everything about integrative cancer treatment? How does it access our specific knowledge?"

"That's where things get interesting," Andreas replied, his eyes lighting up with excitement. "We're using something called a vector database, specifically Pinecone. When we talk about knowledge in AI, we're dealing with 'chunks' of information. These chunks could be sentences, paragraphs, or even entire documents. What we do is convert these chunks into vectors— basically, mathematical representations of the information. It's like turning words into numbers that the AI can understand and work with."

"And Pinecone stores these vectors?" Dr. Dean asked, leaning forward.

"Exactly," Andreas nodded. "Think of Pinecone as a massive library, but instead of books on shelves, it has vectors. When someone asks Cancerase GPT a question, the AI doesn't just guess. It goes through Pinecone, looking for the most relevant chunks of information. It's like flipping through the pages of a book to find the exact section you need."

Dr. Dean was starting to see the picture. "So, it's like having a super-fast research assistant that can find the right information instantly?"

"Exactly!" Andreas said, grinning. "Once it finds the relevant chunks, those are sent back to the LLM—our ChatGPT-4 model. The model then reads those chunks, understands the context, and generates a response. It can write an expertise on a subject, suggest a therapy, or answer any question related to integrative cancer treatment. It's all about using the right data and asking the right questions."

Dr. Dean was amazed. "And we're doing all this with Python and LangChain?"

Andreas chuckled. "Yep! Python is the programming language that powers a lot of AI and machine learning work because it's flexible and easy to use. LangChain is a library that helps us build language models and connect them with other tools, like databases or APIs. With these tools, we've been able to create a seamless workflow where Cancerase GPT can access vast amounts of information and provide accurate, helpful answers."

He continued, "We also use Amazon AWS services to host our AI model and vector database. AWS provides the computational power we need to run our models efficiently. This means that anyone, anywhere, can access Cancerase GPT through the cloud without needing to install anything on their own computers."

Dr. Dean was impressed. "That sounds powerful. But how did we train the AI on all those scientific articles and integrative cancer treatments?"

Andreas explained, "We trained Cancerase GPT by feeding it thousands of scientific articles, research papers, and clinical studies on integrative cancer treatment. This training process involved using machine learning techniques to help the AI recognize patterns, understand complex medical terminology, and learn how different treatments interact with various types of cancer. We didn't just throw all the information at it; we carefully curated and annotated the data to make sure the AI could truly understand and use it effectively."

"And now," Andreas continued, "because it's trained on such a rich dataset, Cancerase GPT isn't just giving generic advice. It can tailor its responses to the specific needs of a patient, suggest innovative treatment combinations, or even recommend new nutritional blends that complement other therapies. It's like having a team of integrative medicine experts available 24/7."

Dr. Dean leaned back in his chair, clearly impressed. "This is incredible, Andreas. We've created something that could genuinely change how people approach cancer treatment."

Andreas smiled, feeling a mix of pride and relief. "That's the goal, Dr. Dean. We want to give everyone access to this knowledge—doctors, patients, families. Cancerase GPT isn't just an AI; it's a bridge to a new way of understanding and treating cancer. And the best part? We're giving it away for free. It's our gift to the world, a tool that could help anyone, anywhere, find the best possible care."

Dr. Dean nodded, feeling a deep sense of satisfaction. "We've done something truly remarkable here, Andreas. We've taken the best of what both of us know—medicine and technology— and created something that can make a real difference."

Andreas agreed. "And this is just the beginning. As more data comes in, as more research is done, Cancerase GPT will continue to learn and grow. It's a living, evolving tool that will only get better with time. We're part of the first experiment on this planet where AI is used to democratize medical knowledge. And that's something worth celebrating."

As they sat in the IV room, surrounded by the steady hum of machines, Andreas and Dr. Dean realized they had not only built a groundbreaking AI but had also forged a new path forward in the fight against cancer. Together, they had created a tool that could change the world—one answer, one patient, one treatment at a time.

Chapter 4: Dr. Dean's Crash Course on Integrative Cancer Treatment

"True wisdom is found where curiosity meets experience. Whether in medicine or technology, the greatest breakthroughs come from those willing to learn, adapt, and see the world through a new lens." Andreas Kazmierczak

The IV room had become a classroom of sorts for Andreas and Dr. Dean. With Andreas having explained the complexities of AI and machine learning, it was now Dr. Dean's turn to share his wealth of knowledge on integrative cancer treatment. Dr. Dean, a seasoned expert in holistic health, was eager to teach Andreas, but little did he know that his AI engineer friend had a knack for taking things quite literally.

"Alright, Andreas," Dr. Dean began, setting aside his papers, "today I'm going to teach you about the integrative methods we use in cancer treatment—nutrition, herbal remedies, and the whole spectrum of natural therapies. These treatments work together to support the body's natural healing processes."

Andreas nodded enthusiastically. "I'm ready, Dr. Dean! Hit me with the knowledge!"

Dr. Dean chuckled. "Let's start with something simple. One of the most powerful natural anticancer agents is turmeric. It contains curcumin, which has remarkable anti-inflammatory and antioxidant properties. In fact, some studies suggest that it can help prevent cancer cells from growing and even induce apoptosis—which means it helps them self-destruct."

Andreas looked puzzled. "Wait, so we're fighting cancer with curry powder? Should we just open an Indian restaurant and call it a day?"

Dr. Dean laughed. "Not exactly, Andreas. While turmeric is a key ingredient in Indian cuisine, the amounts used in food aren't always enough for therapeutic effects. That's why we use curcumin extracts in high doses—but hey, if you want to eat more curry, I'm not going to stop you."

Andreas furrowed his brow. "So, you're saying that India has lower cancer rates partly because turmeric has been a daily part of their diet for centuries?"

Dr. Dean smirked. "Well, let's just say their diet gives them a pretty strong advantage. The U.S. has a significantly higher cancer incidence rate than India. According to the Global Cancer Observatory (GLOBOCAN), the cancer incidence rate in the U.S. is about 350-400 cases per 100,000 people, whereas in India, it is around 100-150 cases per 100,000 people. The anti-inflammatory effects of turmeric, combined with their plant-rich diets, certainly contribute to lower cancer rates compared to the typical Western diet, which is loaded with processed food and inflammation-triggering ingredients."

Andreas nodded slowly, clearly trying to follow along. "Got it. So, turmeric is like the body's secret spice shield against cancer? Like an ancient, golden force field?"

Dr. Dean chuckled. "That's one way to look at it. The curcumin in turmeric targets cancer cells while leaving healthy cells unharmed. Think of it as a precision-guided spice missile."

Andreas grinned. "So, if I start eating enough turmeric, will I turn into a glowing golden warrior immune to disease?"

Dr. Dean rolled his eyes. "Not quite. But it will definitely help reduce chronic inflammation, which is one of the root causes of cancer. The key is balance—using turmeric as part of a well-rounded approach that includes other anticancer foods and treatments."

Andreas perked up. "Plant-based? So, like eating a lot of vegetables? Should I be grazing on grass like a cow?"

Dr. Dean chuckled. "Not exactly. We're talking about a diverse diet rich in antioxidants and phytonutrients. Think of it as eating the rainbow, but instead of a pot of gold at the end, you get a healthier, stronger body."

Andreas gave a thumbs-up. "Alright, so more turmeric, fewer burgers. Got it. But can we still have chocolate? Asking for a friend."

Dr. Dean smirked. "Dark chocolate, in moderation, is fine. It's actually a good source of antioxidants. But we're focusing on whole foods that nourish the body."

Andreas grinned. "So, dark chocolate turmeric curry it is!"

Dr. Dean shook his head, laughing. "You've got a lot to learn, Andreas. Let's talk about herbal remedies next. Turmeric is just one part of a broader integrative treatment strategy. We also use green tea, medicinal mushrooms, and other powerful natural compounds."

Andreas raised an eyebrow. "So, we're turning cancer patients into walking spice racks?"

Dr. Dean laughed. "No, Andreas. It's about using the right natural compounds in a therapeutic way. We combine these approaches to create a synergistic effect, where each treatment enhances the power of the others."

Andreas thought for a moment, then asked, "So, it's like building the ultimate Indian feast, but instead of feeding your belly, it's feeding your immune system?"

Dr. Dean chuckled, shaking his head. "In a way, yes. But it's not just about mixing things together; it's about understanding how each element interacts with the others and with the patient's unique biology. We tailor the treatments to each individual."

Andreas nodded, finally catching on. "Ah, I see. It's like coding— you have to write the right script to get the desired outcome."

Dr. Dean smiled, "Exactly, Andreas. It's all about balance and precision, just like your work with AI."

By the end of their session, Andreas had a much better understanding of integrative cancer treatment, even if his interpretations were a bit humorous. Dr. Dean was pleased with the progress and couldn't help but appreciate Andreas's enthusiasm and unique way of grasping concepts.

"Andreas," Dr. Dean said, patting him on the back, "I have to hand it to you. You might be a bit of a dilettante in the world of medicine, but you're catching on fast. And more importantly, you're bringing a fresh perspective to all this."

Andreas grinned. "Thanks, Dr. Dean. Who knew fighting cancer would involve so much turmeric and curry?"

Dr. Dean laughed. "Well, there's a lot more to it, but I think you're starting to get the hang of it. And remember, just like with coding AI, it's all about continuous learning and improvement."

Andreas nodded, feeling grateful for the crash course in integrative cancer treatment. "You're right, Dr. Dean. And maybe, just maybe, with Cancerase GPT, we can make all this knowledge accessible to everyone, so they don't have to take a crash course like I did."

Dr. Dean smiled warmly. "That's the goal, Andreas. To make this knowledge available to everyone, in a way that's easy to understand and apply. Together, we're creating something that could change the way cancer is treated forever."

And with that, the two unlikely partners continued their work, determined to bring the best of medicine and technology together for the benefit of all. And as they did, they couldn't help but laugh at the journey that had brought them here—a doctor and an engineer, united in their fight against cancer, one turmeric latte, one AI model, and one spice blend at a time.

Chapter 5: Rethinking Chemotherapy

"The best treatments aren't always the most aggressive but the most intelligent. By starving cancer before striking, using lower chemotherapy doses, and supporting the immune system, we can fight smarter—not harder. Healing should not come at the cost of the body's strength, but by working with it." Andreas Kazmierczak

Andreas sat across from Dr. Dean in the IV room, the low hum of machines filling the space. The discussion of alternative cancer treatments had opened Andreas' mind to new possibilities, but one question still lingered.

"What if all of these repurposed drugs and IV therapies don't work?" Andreas asked, his voice steady but filled with curiosity. "Would you then recommend chemotherapy?"

Dr. Dean leaned back in his chair, nodding slowly. "Yes, Andreas. But not in the way it's commonly administered today."

Andreas furrowed his brow. "What do you mean? I thought chemotherapy was pretty standard—high doses aimed at killing the cancer."

Dr. Dean sighed. "That's the problem. When chemotherapy was first introduced, doctors used it with extreme caution. They started with very low doses and carefully monitored the patient's response, increasing it only as necessary. But over time, the approach changed. Now, chemotherapy is given in massive doses, pushing the patient to the brink of survival, just to ensure the cancer is killed."

Andreas frowned. "But if the patient barely survives the treatment, isn't that counterproductive?"

Dr. Dean nodded. "Exactly. That's why I use an older method— one that's far more effective and significantly less damaging."

Andreas leaned forward. "What's the difference?"

Dr. Dean's eyes gleamed with enthusiasm. "It all starts with sugar. Cancer cells thrive on glucose; they have ten times more sugar receptors than normal cells. If you deprive them of sugar, they become desperate—starving for energy. That's when we strike."

Andreas raised an eyebrow. "How do you deprive cancer cells of sugar?"

"We first drastically lower the patient's blood sugar levels before administering chemotherapy," Dr. Dean explained. "When glucose levels drop significantly, cancer cells become hyperactive, desperately searching for any available sugar. At this point, instead of delivering a full dose of chemotherapy, we administer only 10% of the standard amount. Because the cancer is in a vulnerable state, it absorbs the chemotherapy far more efficiently, making a lower dose just as effective as traditional full-strength treatment.

After giving the 10% chemotherapy dose, we then have the patient eat or provide a sugar-water solution. This surge in blood sugar acts like a smart bomb, carrying the chemotherapy straight into the cancer cells—much like a Trojan horse, tricking the cancer into absorbing the very agent that will destroy it.

This approach is known as metronomic low-dose chemotherapy. It originated from tests that revealed its ability to induce a low-dose 'coma' effect on cancer cells, slowing their metabolism and reducing the formation of new blood vessels. This, in turn, lessens the spread of metastases. Unlike traditional high-dose chemotherapy, which can stimulate circulating cancer stem cells and contribute to further metastasis, metronomic chemotherapy avoids this risk while maintaining effectiveness against the tumor."

Andreas was stunned. "So, you're saying that by starving the cancer first, you can use a fraction of the normal chemotherapy dose and still achieve the same results?"

Dr. Dean nodded. "Exactly. And not only does it work better, but it also spares the patient from the extreme side effects of high-dose chemotherapy."

Andreas exhaled. "That sounds revolutionary. Why isn't this standard practice?"

Dr. Dean smirked knowingly. "Because it doesn't sell enough drugs. Pharmaceutical companies make billions from chemotherapy medications. If oncologists started using only 10% of the standard dose, profits would plummet. That's why most doctors don't use this method—it's not lucrative."

Andreas shook his head in disbelief. "That's infuriating. People are suffering when there's a better way."

Dr. Dean's expression grew serious. "It gets worse. Traditional chemotherapy also destroys the immune system. A patient already weakened by cancer is then hit with a treatment that wipes out their body's natural defenses. That's why so many people relapse or succumb to infections during treatment."

Andreas clenched his fists. "So, what's the solution?"

"We support the immune system during chemotherapy,"

Dr. Dean said firmly. "While conventional oncology ignores immune health, we use supplements, IV therapies, and medications to keep the immune system strong throughout treatment. That way, the body can continue fighting alongside the chemo, rather than being devastated by it."

Andreas sat back, absorbing everything. "So, lower the sugar, use a minimal dose of chemotherapy, and support the immune system. It sounds like common sense."

Dr. Dean smiled. "Common sense isn't always common in medicine, Andreas."

Andreas nodded, his mind racing with possibilities. This wasn't just about finding better treatments—it was about changing the entire approach to cancer care. And with Cancerase GPT, they could bring these ideas to light, empowering patients and doctors alike with knowledge that could save lives.

As the IV machine continued its steady hum, Andreas felt a renewed sense of purpose. They were not just fighting cancer— they were fighting for a better way to heal.

Dr. Dean leaned in slightly, his voice growing more serious. "You know, Andreas, low-dose genomically targeted chemotherapy is starting to be used more frequently now. The reason is simple: fewer side effects, better patient compliance, and, ultimately, better outcomes. In my opinion, it's the future."

Andreas raised an eyebrow. "Genomically targeted chemotherapy? What do you mean by that?"

Dr. Dean nodded. "Well, we start with a complete evaluation of the patient. We assess their DNA, RNA, and genetic transcription to get a full understanding of their unique cancer profile. We look at how their cancer cells are behaving, how they're mutating, and what their genetic weaknesses are."

Andreas leaned forward, interested. "So, it's not just about a one-size-fits-all chemotherapy plan?"

"Exactly," Dr. Dean replied. "We take a much more personalized approach. After we've analyzed their genetic makeup, we look at the patient's circulating cancer stem cells or even their circulating DNA. We send these samples to specialized labs to get a baseline before we even think about starting treatment."

Andreas nodded. "That's incredible. But how do you know which chemotherapy will be most effective?"

"Through chemo-sensitivity testing," Dr. Dean explained. "We collect either blood or tissue samples from the patient and perform tests in vitro. These tests show us exactly which chemotherapies will be most effective for that individual patient. We get the results back in percentages, and from there, we combine different chemotherapies to create a synergistic blend that targets the cancer on multiple fronts."

Andreas was amazed. "So, instead of just blasting the cancer with high doses of one drug, you use a combination of lower doses to hit the cancer from different angles?"

"Exactly," Dr. Dean said with a grin. "The goal is to kill the cancer using different pathways, all while minimizing damage to the body—especially to vital organs like the bone marrow, brain, and other critical systems."

Andreas sat back, trying to process it all. "That sounds like a much more efficient and humane approach."

Dr. Dean nodded. "It's a blend of science and common sense. And we're not just focused on the chemotherapy itself. We also test for natural substances—things like medicinal herbs, compounds, and nutrients—because they can be just as effective when used in combination with the right drugs."

"Wow," Andreas said, still stunned. "That sounds like a complete system of care."

"It is," Dr. Dean agreed. "But there's more. We also evaluate the patient's immune system in great detail. We look at markers that most doctors don't even consider—markers for inflammation, toxins, methylation, heavy metals, and even infections. If any of these are out of balance, they could be contributing to the patient's mitochondrial dysfunction, making it harder for them to fight cancer."

Andreas sat forward again. "So, you're treating the patient as a whole, not just the cancer."

Dr. Dean smiled. "Exactly. It's about understanding the root causes of their illness, and addressing those along with the cancer. Once we have all the lab data and evaluations, we can formulate a completely personalized, genomic, and targeted treatment plan."

"Does diet play a role in this?" Andreas asked.

"Absolutely," Dr. Dean replied. "Once we have all the data, we put the patient on a ketogenic, plant-based organic diet. This diet helps to create an alkaline environment in the body, which is critical for preventing the cancer from spreading and metastasizing. We also make sure the patient is exercising and practicing mind-body relaxation techniques to help them handle the stress of the treatment. And sleep hygiene is crucial as well."

Andreas nodded, feeling more and more inspired. "It sounds like the treatment is ongoing—something that needs constant monitoring and adjustment."

"Exactly," Dr. Dean agreed. "We periodically monitor the patient by evaluating their circulating DNA, cancer stem cells, and using PET scans, MRIs, and CAT scans. It's a continuous process, and we follow up with them long-term. Most of our patients stay with us for life, continuing to do well."

Andreas could see the bigger picture now—a truly integrated approach that was about much more than just treating cancer. It was about empowering the patient to take control of their health, using cutting-edge science combined with holistic care to heal their body, mind, and spirit.

Dr. Dean's expression softened as he shared a personal story. "In 2006, my father was diagnosed with transitional cell bladder cancer. He was receiving standard chemotherapy in Philadelphia, but he wasn't doing well at all. I was at a conference in Germany when I heard a lecture about tracking cancer cells in the blood and finding out what chemo would actually work. I decided to have that test performed on my father."

Andreas looked intrigued. "So, what happened?"

Dr. Dean smiled. "It turned out my father was receiving the wrong chemotherapy. After the test results came back, I changed his treatment to the right one. It was low-dose chemotherapy, tailored specifically for his cancer. The results were incredible. He went on to live into his mid-90s without any more cancer. That was the first case I cured with low-dose chemotherapy."

Andreas' eyes widened. "That's amazing."

Dr. Dean's face lit up with pride. "It was a turning point in my career. I realized the power of genomically targeted, low-dose chemotherapy. It was effective, it spared the body, and it gave patients their lives back."

Andreas felt a deep sense of purpose. This was more than just a treatment—it was a revolution in cancer care. And with Cancerase GPT, they had the chance to change the future of medicine, one patient at a time.

Dr. Silver had always believed that cancer treatment needed to evolve beyond the traditional methods. After years of research and clinical trials, he discovered a groundbreaking approach— one that combined the power of natural products with low-dose metronomic targeted chemotherapy. It was a combination that would change the way cancer was treated and give patients a fighting chance without the debilitating side effects.

He had spent years studying the interactions between various natural compounds and chemotherapy drugs. Through his research, he identified several natural products that showed incredible promise when used in combination with chemotherapy. Compounds like curcumin, artesunate, resveratrol, and many others had all demonstrated synergistic effects that enhanced the efficacy of chemotherapy while minimizing the toxic burden on the body.

Curcumin, for instance, known for its anti-inflammatory properties, could inhibit tumor growth and prevent cancer cells from metastasizing. Artesunate, derived from the sweet wormwood plant, was shown to target cancer cells more effectively, making it a powerful addition to chemotherapy. Resveratrol, found in grapes and berries, was another powerful ally, offering antioxidant protection and slowing cancer cell growth.

When combined with chemotherapy, these natural products didn't just sit idly by—they amplified the chemotherapy's ability to target cancer cells, making the treatment more effective without the need for high, toxic doses. This allowed Dr. Silver to use much lower doses of chemotherapy, which meant far fewer side effects for his patients.

The result? Patients felt better. Many of them reported feeling more energetic, experiencing fewer bouts of nausea, and avoiding the debilitating hair loss and fatigue that usually accompanied traditional high-dose chemotherapy. In fact, most of Dr. Silver's patients—who were accustomed to the harsh side effects of standard treatment—were often surprised at how well they felt. Some even requested that he increase their chemotherapy doses, believing that more was better.

Dr. Silver would smile and remind them that the goal wasn't to bombard the body with more toxins but to strike a balance— using the right dose of chemotherapy alongside natural compounds that supported the body's healing processes. He had learned that less truly could be more, and in many cases, his patients thrived because of it.

His approach had become a new standard in his clinic, one that combined the best of modern medicine with the ancient wisdom of nature. And while the rest of the medical world slowly caught up to this more integrative approach, Dr. Silver was already seeing the incredible impact it had on his patients' lives. Cancer care had been transformed, not by increasing the dose of poison, but by using smarter, synergistic treatments that allowed the body to heal itself.

Chapter 6: Decoding Vitamin C - Dr. Dean's Lesson for Andreas

"Healing, like knowledge, is about balance—too little and it's ineffective, too much and it overwhelms. Whether in medicine or technology, the key to progress is understanding how to harness power without losing control." Andreas Kazmierczak

Another day, another IV session in their familiar room at the clinic. Andreas was getting used to the routine by now, his laptop balanced on his knees as he continued to tweak Cancerase GPT. He had been feeling a little off lately—some headaches, a bit of nausea—but nothing too alarming. Today, though, Dr. Dean had something different in mind for their usual chat.

"Andreas, I want to explain something important about one of the treatments we're using," Dr. Dean said, pulling up a chair next to him. "You've been getting high doses of Vitamin C intravenously, and I think it's time you understood exactly how it works."

Andreas looked up from his laptop, intrigued. "Sure, Dr. Dean. I know Vitamin C is good for you, but what's special about this high-dose treatment?"

Dr. Dean smiled. "Well, let me break it down for you. Normally, when people think of Vitamin C, they think of it as an antioxidant—a good thing that helps protect your cells from damage. And that's true, but when we use it in these extremely high doses—like 100 grams—things change."

Andreas's eyes widened. "100 grams? How much is that in oranges?"

Dr. Dean chuckled. "Good question. It's roughly the equivalent of thousands of oranges. Imagine trying to eat hundreds of boxes of oranges in one sitting. That's the amount of Vitamin C we're talking about here, and no human could ever digest that much by eating fruit. But when we administer it intravenously, it bypasses the digestive system and goes straight into your bloodstream."

Andreas scratched his head, trying to wrap his mind around it. "Okay, so we're talking about a massive dose. But what does that do?"

"That's where it gets interesting," Dr. Dean continued. "In such high doses, Vitamin C acts as a pro-oxidant rather than an antioxidant. It's like flipping a switch. Instead of just protecting cells, it starts producing hydrogen peroxide in your body."

Andreas blinked, confused. "Hydrogen peroxide? Isn't that the stuff you use to clean cuts?"

"Yes, exactly," Dr. Dean said. "But in this context, it plays a different role. The peroxide generated by this high dose of Vitamin C can actually damage cancer cells. Cancer cells are less capable of handling the oxidative stress caused by hydrogen peroxide than healthy cells. So, while the peroxide damages the cancer cells, your healthy cells, which can manage this kind of oxidative stress, remain unharmed."

Andreas leaned back in his chair, processing this new information. "So, it's like using Vitamin C as a targeted missile. It hits the cancer cells hard but leaves the healthy cells alone?"

"Exactly," Dr. Dean nodded. "That's a good way to think about it. But, just like any treatment, there can be side effects. In these high doses, Vitamin C can sometimes cause headaches or nausea because your body is reacting to the large amount of hydrogen peroxide being produced."

Andreas rubbed his temples, thinking about the headaches he'd had recently. "That makes sense. I've definitely felt a bit off during some of these treatments."

Dr. Dean smiled knowingly. "Yes, that's a common side effect. But consider this: the symptoms you're experiencing are relatively mild compared to the harsh side effects of chemotherapy, like severe nausea, fatigue, and hair loss. The goal here is to target the cancer cells without causing too much collateral damage to the rest of your body."

Andreas nodded, though he still looked a bit perplexed. "I get that. But it's a lot to take in. So, we're basically overloading the body with Vitamin C to trigger this peroxide effect?"

Dr. Dean could see Andreas struggling to grasp the concept fully. "Think of it this way, Andreas: it's like feeding your AI system a massive dataset.

If you feed it too much all at once, it could slow down and maybe even cause some 'headaches' for the system as it processes all that information. But if the data is the right kind, it can actually make the AI more efficient and effective at its job."

Andreas's eyes lit up. "Ah, I see! So, Vitamin C in these huge doses is like a big batch of data that's tough to handle, but if processed correctly, it can help achieve a better outcome. It might slow things down temporarily—like giving the AI a lot to chew on—but ultimately, it makes the AI smarter and more effective."

Dr. Dean laughed. "Exactly! You've got it. The headaches and nausea are like the system slowing down a bit while it adjusts to the new load. But once your body processes the peroxide, it can get back to fighting the cancer cells effectively, just like an AI getting back to its task after digesting a big data dump."

Andreas grinned, clearly pleased with his analogy. "So, Vitamin C is like data in AI. It might cause some temporary discomfort, but in the end, it's helping the system—my body—work better against the cancer. And the side effects are much more manageable than traditional chemotherapy."

"Precisely," Dr. Dean said, nodding. "We're using these integrative treatments to make your body more efficient at targeting the cancer, just like we use data to make AI more intelligent.

The key is finding the right balance and understanding how each treatment works with your body's unique system."

Andreas leaned back in his chair, feeling a new sense of clarity. "That actually makes a lot of sense. Thanks for breaking it down for me, Dr. Dean. I guess even AI engineers can learn a thing or two about how the body works."

Dr. Dean chuckled. "We're all learning, Andreas. And the more we understand about how these treatments work, the better we can use them to help people. Whether it's through AI or Vitamin C, the goal is the same: to give people the best chance at beating cancer and living healthy, full lives."

Andreas smiled, grateful for the explanation and the newfound understanding. "And with Cancerase GPT and these integrative treatments, we're giving people more than just a fighting chance. We're giving them hope."

Dr. Dean nodded. "Exactly. And that's something worth fighting for, every single day."

With that, they returned to their work, each more committed than ever to their mission. In their own ways—one with code and algorithms, the other with medicine and care—they were forging a new path forward in the fight against cancer. And together, they knew they could make a real difference.

Chapter 7: Andreas' Long Journey to Dr. Dean

*"True healing begins when we dare to look beyond convention.
The greatest breakthroughs happen when we trust wisdom over
fear, embrace knowledge over dogma, and seek care that nourishes
both body and spirit."* Andreas Kazmierczak

Andreas' battle with cancer began two years before he met Dr.
Dean. His life took a drastic turn when he was diagnosed with
prostate cancer, receiving a Gleason score of 9. The Gleason
score is a system used by doctors to assess the aggressiveness
of prostate cancer based on how the cancer cells look under
a microscope. Scores range from 2 to 10, with higher scores
indicating more aggressive cancer that is more likely to spread.
A score of 9 meant Andreas' cancer was highly aggressive and
had a significant risk of spreading quickly.

To combat this, Andreas underwent a radical prostatectomy, a
major surgical procedure in which the entire prostate gland and
some surrounding tissues are removed. This surgery is often
recommended when the cancer is believed to be confined to the
prostate gland, aiming to remove the cancer entirely and prevent
it from spreading to other parts of the body.
Initially, after the surgery, Andreas was informed by his doctors
that his prostate-specific antigen (PSA) levels had dropped to
undetectable levels, suggesting that there were no longer any
detectable cancer cells in his body.

This period of low or undetectable PSA is often referred to as
being in remission, but it is critical to understand that it does
not guarantee the cancer is gone permanently. In many cases,
particularly with aggressive cancers, the disease can return.

Unfortunately, Andreas' relief was short-lived. After several months, his PSA levels began to rise again, signaling a recurrence. A recurrence is when cancer returns after a period of being undetectable or stable. In Andreas' case, this meant that despite the surgery, cancer cells had remained in his body and had begun to grow again. The news was a heavy blow. He had hoped that the surgery would be the end of his cancer journey, but now he was facing the terrifying reality that his battle was far from over.

Desperate for a solution, Andreas began to explore alternative and integrative cancer care, which combines conventional treatments like surgery and chemotherapy with complementary approaches such as nutritional therapy, vitamins, and mind-body practices. He was eager to begin this new path under the guidance of Dr. Dean, an expert in integrative oncology known for his holistic approach to cancer care.

However, before he could start, Andreas received conflicting advice from several conventional doctors. One radiologist made a particularly dismissive comment, saying, "Instead of pursuing integrative cancer care, you'd be better off taking a vacation to Mexico." Andreas was stunned by this suggestion, which seemed like a thinly veiled expression of hostility toward integrative cancer care. The comment was not just impractical but felt like a deliberate critique of Andreas' desire to pursue a more holistic approach. How could he think of a vacation when he was so weak from the radiation treatments that he could barely manage a short walk in his own yard?

Another doctor, a traditional oncologist, warned him against taking Vitamin C, claiming that it could "feed the cancer." This advice contradicted much of the research Andreas had read, which indicated that high-dose Vitamin C, especially intravenously, could act as a pro-oxidant in the body, creating an environment that was hostile to cancer cells.

Yet another physician told him that during radiation therapy, he should avoid taking any vitamins at all, stating that they could interfere with the treatment. This advice seemed both counterintuitive and illogical, considering that many vitamins and nutrients are essential for maintaining overall health and could potentially help the body cope with the side effects of radiation.

Confused and overwhelmed by these conflicting opinions, Andreas decided to follow the conventional medical advice. He began a grueling regimen of 40 pelvic radiation sessions, hoping it would be the answer to his cancer's recurrence. However, this decision proved to be a mistake. The radiation severely damaged his immune system, leaving him incredibly weak and unable to perform even the simplest daily tasks.

Walking became a challenge, and his energy levels were completely depleted. The idea of a vacation now seemed not just impractical but absurd—a vacation when he had no immune system left? A vacation when he could barely stand?

Disheartened and feeling betrayed by the traditional medical approach, Andreas knew he needed a different strategy. He reached out to Dr. Dean, hoping for a solution that went beyond the limited scope of conventional medicine.

When Andreas met Dr. Dean, he was immediately struck by the doctor's calm demeanor and profound empathy. Unlike the other doctors, Dr. Dean didn't criticize the previous treatments or question Andreas' decisions.

He listened carefully and focused on what could be done moving forward. Dr. Dean's approach was refreshing and empowering. He offered hope without making unrealistic promises and focused on integrating all possible methods to support Andreas' health and fight the cancer.

Dr. Dean explained that his approach to integrative cancer care involved combining the best of conventional and alternative therapies. He outlined a comprehensive plan that included high-dose Vitamin C to exploit its pro-oxidant effects, targeted nutritional supplements, a carefully designed diet, and various mind-body practices to help rebuild Andreas' immune system and overall health.

Under Dr. Dean's guidance, Andreas began to implement this new plan. The effects were transformative. Slowly but steadily, Andreas' strength began to return, and his immune system started to recover. The cancer, which had seemed ready to spread further, began to show signs of retreating. Andreas' energy improved, his outlook brightened, and he finally felt like he was on the right path.

Dr. Dean's commitment to patient care and his willingness to explore all treatment avenues made all the difference for Andreas. Unlike the other doctors who had given him conflicting and often discouraging advice, Dr. Dean approached his case with an open mind and a focus on healing. He was not concerned with maintaining rigid treatment protocols or following outdated practices. Instead, he prioritized Andreas' well-being and tailored his approach to meet his unique needs.

In the end, Andreas realized that Dr. Dean was more than just a doctor; he was a healer in the truest sense. He was someone who wasn't afraid to think outside the box, who had the courage to challenge the status quo, and who dedicated himself to providing the best possible care for his patients.

Through his innovative approach to integrative cancer care, Dr. Dean had saved Andreas' life, giving him hope and healing when all seemed lost. For Andreas, Dr. Dean was not just a physician but a true hero—someone who cared deeply about his patients and was willing to do whatever it took to help them heal.

Dr. Dean's dedication to integrative cancer care demonstrated that true healing is possible when doctors are willing to look beyond the conventional and embrace a more holistic, patient-centered approach.

Chapter 8: Cancer for Sale - Navigating the Business of Fear

"Fear is the most profitable currency in medicine, but true healing is never for sale. The right path is not found in desperation, but in knowledge, integrity, and the courage to seek what truly works."
Andreas Kazmierczak

Andreas never imagined that receiving a cancer diagnosis would come with an avalanche of unsolicited advice, miracle cures, and aggressive sales tactics. But the moment his diagnosis became known, his phone wouldn't stop ringing. Messages flooded his inbox. Some came from well-meaning friends suggesting obscure treatments, but most were from people he had never met—practitioners, supplement companies, alternative healers—all promising one thing: a cure.

At first, Andreas thought it was a coincidence. But as he picked up the calls, a chilling pattern emerged. One supposed doctor, whom he had never seen in person, spent less than five minutes on the phone with him before making a bold declaration:

"You need immediate blood cleansing, special supplements, and absolutely no conventional treatment. I can set you up with a protocol for $10,000. Time is of the essence."

Andreas was stunned. How could this man—who knew nothing about his case, had never seen his medical reports, and had no idea about his specific cancer type—confidently prescribe an expensive treatment over the phone?

And that was just the beginning.

There were others—people selling $10 bottles of "miracle water," promising that cancer could be flushed out of his system with a special alkaline diet, energy healing, or secret herbal blends. On the other end of the spectrum, the pharmaceutical industry stood with its own set of tactics—pushing newly approved drugs with astronomical price tags, ensuring doctors received handsome commissions for prescribing them. The system was a machine, a massive business feeding on the desperation of those who were simply looking for a chance to survive.

Andreas found himself drowning in information, sales pitches, and fear. Who could he trust? Was there even a right path?

He had always believed in science, in data, in logic. But cancer was different. It didn't come with a clear instruction manual. Everyone had an opinion, everyone had a treatment, but no one was asking the most important question:

"Does it actually work?"

The deeper he went, the more he realized that cancer treatment was not just about medicine—it was a maze of fear, business, and human vulnerability. Patients were selling their homes, liquidating their savings, doing anything to grasp at a chance for survival.

Andreas needed clarity. He needed guidance. He needed someone who wasn't just another salesman in a white coat.

And then, he stood in front of Dr. Dean.

For the first time since his diagnosis, Andreas felt something other than fear—he felt grounded. Dr. Dean wasn't pushing a miracle cure or offering a one-size-fits-all treatment plan. He wasn't interested in pharmaceutical commissions or alternative treatments without real merit. Instead, he listened. Really listened.

"Let's look at everything," Dr. Dean said. "Your medical reports, your lifestyle, your treatment options. We take what works—conventional, integrative, whatever has evidence—and we create a real strategy. This isn't about selling hope. It's about giving you the best chance."

In that moment, Andreas realized what had been missing in the sea of confusion: a doctor who cared more about the patient than the paycheck.

Dr. Dean was a rare breed—an experienced physician who understood both conventional and integrative medicine, who didn't blindly follow pharmaceutical incentives, and who had no interest in selling false hope. He wasn't just a doctor; he was a guide through the chaos.

With each visit, Andreas felt his fear loosening its grip. There was finally a clear path forward—a structured plan based on evidence, experience, and a genuine commitment to healing. And that, more than any overpriced treatment or miracle cure, was what every cancer patient truly needed.

"We need more doctors like him," Andreas thought. Doctors who put patients before profit, who understand that healing is not just about medicine, but about trust, compassion, and wisdom.

And with that realization, he took his first real step toward not just fighting cancer—but truly understanding how to heal.

Chapter 9: Andreas and the Apigenin Treatment

"Nature holds powerful secrets, but harnessing them requires precision. The right dose, the right method, and the right knowledge turn simple remedies into life-changing treatments."
Andreas Kazmierczak

Andreas sat across from Dr. Dean in the clinic, eyeing the small bottle of supplements that Dr. Dean had just handed him. "So, what's this new miracle cure?" Andreas asked, turning the bottle in his hands. He read the label: Apigenin – 100 mg.

"Apigenin," Dr. Dean replied with a grin, "It's a powerful natural compound that's been shown to help in the fight against cancer. You'll be taking 100 mg daily."

Andreas furrowed his brow, trying to recall where he had heard that name before. "Apigenin… wait a minute. Isn't that the stuff found in chamomile tea?"

Dr. Dean nodded. "Exactly! Chamomile tea is one of the most common sources of apigenin. But what's in this bottle is a bit more concentrated."

Andreas chuckled, a playful skepticism in his voice. "So, you're telling me I'm going to beat cancer with chamomile tea? I drink a cup of that stuff every night to help me sleep! Should I have been upping my dosage all along?"

Dr. Dean laughed at Andreas' reaction. "Well, if you're planning to cure cancer with chamomile tea, you'd need to be drinking about a hundred cups a day to get close to the amount of apigenin you need. And that, my friend, would probably ruin your kidneys and leave you with a very full bladder every half hour!"

Andreas burst out laughing, picturing himself trying to guzzle down an endless stream of chamomile tea. "A hundred cups a day? I'd spend more time in the bathroom than actually fighting cancer!"

"Exactly!" Dr. Dean said, still chuckling. "That's why we're using a concentrated supplement. Apigenin, in high doses, can help inhibit the growth of cancer cells. It's known for its anti-inflammatory and antioxidant properties, but in large amounts, it also promotes apoptosis, which is the process of programmed cell death that helps get rid of damaged cells, like cancer cells."

Andreas' laughter faded into curiosity. "So, how exactly does it work? I mean, what makes it so special?"

Dr. Dean leaned back in his chair, adopting a more serious tone. "Apigenin is a flavonoid, which is a type of plant compound found in many fruits and vegetables. It's been studied for its potential to slow down or stop the growth of cancer cells. It works in several ways: it can induce apoptosis, like I mentioned, but it also inhibits cell proliferation, which means it can prevent cancer cells from multiplying. Additionally, it's been found to interfere with certain proteins and enzymes that cancer cells use to protect themselves and grow."

Andreas nodded, starting to see the potential. "So, it's not just about drinking a lot of tea, huh?"

Dr. Dean smiled. "No, it's a bit more scientific than that. The amount of apigenin in a single cup of chamomile tea is very low. You'd have to drink a truly ridiculous amount of tea to get the same therapeutic effect. That's why we use the concentrated form in supplement form. This way, you're getting a powerful dose that can actually make a difference in fighting the cancer."

Andreas rubbed his chin thoughtfully. "And here I was, thinking I could just load up on chamomile and call it a day. Shows what I know!"

Dr. Dean chuckled again. "You're not alone. A lot of people think that because something is found in a common food or drink, it's easy to get the right amount through diet alone. But in reality, therapeutic doses of compounds like apigenin require much higher concentrations than what we'd get from regular food or drinks. That's why supplements are so important in integrative cancer care—they allow us to harness the full potential of these natural compounds in a way that's actually effective."

Andreas smiled, feeling more confident about the new treatment plan. "Alright, I'm sold. I'll take the 100 mg of apigenin. Just promise me I won't have to drink my weight in chamomile tea to make this work!"

Dr. Dean laughed. "Deal. Stick to the supplements, and you'll be just fine. And remember, this is just one part of your treatment. We're using every tool we have to give you the best possible chance."

Andreas nodded, feeling a renewed sense of determination. He might not be curing his cancer with chamomile tea, but with Dr. Dean's guidance, he was confident he was on the right path.

As Andreas left the clinic, he couldn't help but chuckle to himself, imagining what his life would have been like if he had taken the chamomile tea route. "A hundred cups a day," he muttered with a grin. "I'd need a bigger bathroom."

Chapter 10: Andreas and the Mathematics of Cancer Recurrence

"Numbers tell a story, but only when you ask the right questions. Medicine, like life, is more than statistics—it's about patterns, perspective, and the courage to challenge what doesn't add up."

Andreas Kazmierczak

Andreas sat across from Dr. Dean in the familiar IV room, a smirk playing on his lips. He had a notebook open in front of him, filled with numbers, percentages, and a series of calculations. Dr. Dean was accustomed to Andreas' intellectual curiosity, but today he seemed particularly animated, as if he'd discovered something big.

"Alright, Dr. Dean, I've been doing some thinking," Andreas began, tapping his pen against the notebook. "I've been crunching some numbers about this whole prostate cancer thing, and I think I've stumbled upon a statistical anomaly."

Dr. Dean raised an eyebrow, intrigued. "A statistical anomaly? In cancer treatment?"

"Yes, exactly!" Andreas said, leaning forward with excitement. "Look, I was reading up on the probabilities involved in prostate cancer. The chance of having an enlarged prostate is about 50%. The probability of getting cancer if your prostate is enlarged is around 20%. The chance of having a Gleason score of 9 is roughly 5%. Then, if you do get cancer, the probability of recurrence after surgery is 20%, the recurrence after radiation is also 20%, and the recurrence after hormone therapy is again 20%."

Dr. Dean nodded, trying to follow along. "Alright, I'm with you so far. Those sound like fairly standard statistics."

"Right," Andreas continued, his voice picking up pace. "So, I started thinking, 'What are the odds of all these things happening to the same person?' I mean, I've hit every single one of these terrible milestones. Enlarged prostate, cancer, Gleason score of 9, recurrence after surgery, recurrence after radiation, and now recurrence after hormone therapy. So, I did the math."

Dr. Dean leaned in closer, curious. "And what did you find?"

Andreas grinned. "I multiplied all the probabilities together. 50% for the enlarged prostate, 20% for the cancer, 5% for the Gleason score of 9, and then 20% for each type of recurrence. So, that's 50% times 20% times 5% times 20% times 20% times 20%. Do you know what that comes out to?"

Dr. Dean shook his head. "No idea, but I'm sure you're going to tell me."

Andreas slapped his hand on the notebook. "0.0004%! That's four in a million! According to my calculations, only four out of a million men should have the exact same series of unfortunate events that I've experienced."

Dr. Dean chuckled. "Four in a million? Andreas, you're telling me you're one in a million."

Andreas nodded vigorously. "Exactly! That's what I'm saying. But here's the thing—this can't be right. I know dozens of men in just my area who have had similar recurrences and complications. If my calculations were correct, I'd have to be the unluckiest man in the world, or there's something wrong with these statistics."

Dr. Dean smiled, amused by Andreas' enthusiasm. "So, what's your theory?"

"Well, I ran this through our AI model," Andreas said, now sounding very much like the AI engineer he was. "I asked it to analyze the data, and the AI concluded that the only way my probability could be so low yet so many people are experiencing these recurrences is if the success rates of the conventional therapies are overestimated. The reported success rates must be inflated. If the real success rates were lower, it would match my observations."

Dr. Dean laughed heartily. "So, you're saying the conventional data is, what, a little optimistic?"

"Little? Far too optimistic!" Andreas said, now thoroughly enjoying himself. "The numbers don't add up unless you assume that the success rates of these treatments are far not as high as reported. Maybe they're only a few percentage points better than chance. That would explain why so many of us are ending up with recurrent cancer despite following all the standard protocols."

Dr. Dean chuckled, shaking his head. "I've got to hand it to you, Andreas. Leave it to an AI engineer to analyze cancer treatment like a software bug. But you do have a point. Statistics in medicine are often presented in the best possible light, and recurrence rates can be quite complex. It's not always as straightforward as the numbers make it seem."

Andreas leaned back in his chair, a satisfied grin on his face. "See, I knew there was something off. You can't fool an AI engineer with dodgy statistics. I just needed a bit of logic and some number-crunching to figure it out."

Dr. Dean nodded, still smiling. "And that's why we don't rely solely on statistics. Every patient is unique, and so is every treatment journey. Numbers can help guide us, but they're not the whole story."

Andreas raised his notebook like a trophy. "Well, I'll keep this calculation as a reminder. A reminder that I'm either incredibly unlucky, or I've just uncovered a medical mystery!"

Dr. Dean laughed. "Or maybe a bit of both, Andreas. But either way, I'm glad you're on the case. Keep those calculations coming, and maybe you'll solve the puzzle yet."

Andreas laughed along with Dr. Dean, feeling a sense of accomplishment. He might not have solved the mystery of cancer, but he had certainly brought a bit of humor and perspective to the journey. And in the end, that was just as valuable.

Chapter 11: The Paradox of Mistletoe

"Nature often hides its greatest weapons in its contradictions. What thrives as a parasite in one world can become a healer in another—turning its own aggression into a force for survival."
Andreas Kazmierczak

Andreas sat in the IV room, his mind buzzing with questions as he watched Dr. Dean prepare a new treatment. A small vial labeled "Mistletoe Extract - Pini viscum" sat on the table between them. Andreas leaned forward, curiosity etched on his face. "So, what's this new treatment about, Dr. Dean? Mistletoe? Isn't that the stuff we hang up during Christmas for people to kiss under?"

Dr. Dean chuckled, shaking his head. "Yes, it's the same plant, but we're not using it for holiday decoration. Mistletoe, particularly the type that grows on pine trees, known as Pini viscum, has been used in integrative cancer therapy for years. It contains lectins, which are actually poisons, but in controlled doses, they have a unique ability to stimulate the immune system and target cancer cells."

Andreas raised an eyebrow, intrigued but skeptical. "So, we're using a parasite to fight cancer? How does that even work?"

Dr. Dean nodded. "Exactly. Mistletoe is a semi-parasitic plant that grows on various trees, extracting water and nutrients from its host. But what's fascinating is how it interacts with the human body.

Mistletoe extract can boost the immune response and encourage the body's natural killer cells to attack cancer cells. It's like training your immune system to recognize and fight off cancer more effectively."

Andreas was fascinated by the concept but couldn't help but feel a bit uneasy. "Wait a minute," he said, his mind racing. "Mistletoe is a parasite. It takes over a tree, weakens it, and eventually, both the mistletoe and the tree die. Isn't that... a bit like cancer itself? Cancer grows in the body, takes over, and if left unchecked, it kills its host."

Dr. Dean smiled, appreciating Andreas' insight. "That's a good observation, Andreas. Mistletoe, like cancer, is indeed parasitic in nature. It grows and thrives at the expense of its host. But unlike cancer, when used in controlled doses as a treatment, mistletoe doesn't kill the host. Instead, it seems to provoke a beneficial response."

Andreas leaned back, still pondering the irony. "So, mistletoe and cancer are both aggressive, almost mindlessly so, destroying what they rely on for survival. There's no logic to it. It's like they're programmed to destroy, even if it means their own end. But then, mistletoe somehow becomes a weapon against cancer when used properly?

Dr. Dean nodded again. "Exactly. It's one of those paradoxes in nature. Mistletoe's aggressive characteristics may be the very reason it's effective against cancer. In small, controlled doses, it's almost as if mistletoe is mimicking cancer's aggression, but turning it against the cancer cells instead."

Curious, Andreas decided to ask Cancerase GPT about mistletoe and its properties. He opened his laptop and typed in his query, waiting as the AI processed the information. When the response came back, it was both illuminating and puzzling.

"Mistletoe (Viscum album) has been shown to enhance immune activity, particularly by stimulating natural killer cells. It contains various bioactive compounds, including lectins, which induce apoptosis (cell death) in cancer cells. However, mistletoe's parasitic nature on trees mirrors the destructive behavior of cancer cells within a host organism, suggesting a unique biological parallel."

Andreas read the text aloud and then looked up at Dr. Dean. "So, mistletoe's behavior in nature—its parasitic growth, its tendency to eventually kill its host—mirrors cancer's behavior in the human body.

Yet, when we use mistletoe to treat cancer, it seems to attack the cancer cells rather than the healthy cells. It's like mistletoe recognizes cancer as a competitor and wants to eliminate it. It's as if one aggressive beast is helping us to fight another."

Dr. Dean leaned back in his chair, thoughtful. "That's an interesting way to look at it. Mistletoe is indeed aggressive, but perhaps that's why it's so effective. The immune response it triggers is strong, almost as if the body recognizes mistletoe as a threat and ramps up its defenses, which in turn helps to attack the cancer cells more effectively."

Andreas nodded slowly, piecing it together. "So, it's like mistletoe doesn't like competition. It's a parasite, sure, but when it's introduced into the body, it seems to signal the immune system to treat cancer cells as a hostile force.

It's almost like mistletoe has a 'character' similar to cancer—a desire to dominate and outcompete. In that sense, mistletoe becomes a strange ally, using its aggressive nature to target the cancer's aggression."

Dr. Dean smiled. "You're onto something, Andreas. It's a mysterious story, indeed. Mistletoe, with its unique properties, seems to trigger a profound immune response. Some might even say it's like the mistletoe 'reminds' the immune system how to fight, almost as if it's sounding an alarm."

Andreas pondered this, feeling a deeper sense of wonder. "It's almost like there's more to these cells than just their biology. Mistletoe and cancer both seem to have a kind of 'character' or behavior pattern that's eerily similar. Maybe that's why mistletoe is so effective against cancer—because they understand each other in a way, they're both fighters, but mistletoe is on our side."

Dr. Dean nodded in agreement. "It does make you wonder, doesn't it? There's still so much we don't understand about these natural treatments. The way mistletoe interacts with the body is certainly unique.

Perhaps it's because mistletoe, like cancer, is aggressive and unyielding. When introduced to the body, it doesn't just sit back—it challenges the cancer, provokes the immune system, and creates an environment where the body can fight back more effectively."

Andreas smiled, his curiosity piqued. "It's like a story of one aggressive force combating another. Mistletoe, in its natural state, is a bit of a villain to the trees, but for us, it becomes a hero against cancer. It's fascinating how these parallels exist in nature."

Dr. Dean agreed, his expression thoughtful. "Indeed. It's one of those mysteries that makes medicine so intriguing. Nature has its own way of balancing things out, even if it doesn't always make sense at first glance. But that's why we're here—to explore, to learn, and to use these natural tools in the fight against cancer."

Andreas nodded, feeling a renewed sense of purpose. "Let's see what this mistletoe can do, then. If it's got the character to challenge cancer, then I'm ready to let it help me fight."

With that, Dr. Dean began the mistletoe injection, and Andreas settled back into his chair, ready to face this new chapter in his treatment with a mix of hope and curiosity. The story of mistletoe and its aggressive nature had given him a new perspective on his own battle—one where even the most unlikely allies could make a difference.

Chapter 12: Dr. Dean and the Magic AI Button

"Knowledge isn't just about having the right answers—it's about asking the right questions. The real power of AI isn't automation, but collaboration, where human curiosity meets limitless information." Andreas Kazmierczak

Dr. Dean sat in front of the computer, his glasses perched precariously on the end of his nose, his fingers hovering uncertainly over the keyboard. He had been staring at the screen for a good fifteen minutes, his expression a mix of confusion and curiosity. "So, let me get this straight," he muttered to himself, glancing over at Andreas. "All I need to do is push a button, and this AI, Cancerase GPT, will write a scientific article for me?"

Andreas, who was seated nearby, looked up from his laptop, suppressing a smile. He had explained how Cancerase GPT worked to Dr. Dean several times already, but it seemed that the good doctor still didn't quite get it.

"Not exactly, Dr. Dean," Andreas began, trying to keep his tone patient. "Cancerase GPT isn't like a magic button that just writes an article for you. It's more like a very knowledgeable assistant who needs guidance and direction. You have to ask it the right questions—give it the right prompts—to get the information you need."

Dr. Dean furrowed his brow, clearly not convinced. "But why can't I just tell it to write a scientific article? Isn't it supposed to be intelligent? I thought the whole point of artificial intelligence was that it could do things like this."

Andreas chuckled. "Well, yes and no. Cancerase GPT is intelligent in its way, but it doesn't work like a human brain.

It's not like you press a 'write a scientific article' button, and it magically knows what kind of article you want, what style, what tone, what content… Cancerase GPT needs specific instructions to know what you're looking for."

Dr. Dean still looked skeptical. He leaned forward and pressed a few keys on the keyboard, muttering under his breath, "Alright, Cancerase GPT, write me a scientific article about integrative cancer care. Go."

The cursor blinked on the screen, and then, to Dr. Dean's surprise, a response appeared: "Can you please provide more details on the specific topic, structure, and focus you would like the article to have?"

Dr. Dean groaned in frustration. "See, this is exactly what I mean! I have to do everything myself. It's just like working with people. Why can't this AI just know what I want?"

Andreas laughed, shaking his head. "That's the thing, Dr. Dean. Cancerase GPT isn't a mind reader. It's like when you're working with a specialist—if you want them to give you specific insights, you have to ask specific questions. You wouldn't just say, 'Tell me everything about cancer' and expect them to list every single fact they know. You have to guide them, ask about particular cases, treatments, or scenarios. Cancerase GPT is the same way."

Dr. Dean leaned back in his chair, rubbing his temples. "Alright, fine. I get that. But how do I know what questions to ask? I'm a doctor, not a programmer!"

"That's the art of prompting," Andreas replied, leaning forward to help. "Think of it like a conversation. You ask a question based on what you want to know, and Cancerase GPT responds. Then, based on that answer, you ask another question.

It's interactive. You have to engage with it to pull out the knowledge." Dr. Dean sighed, clearly still frustrated. "So, it's like playing twenty questions with a robot. Why can't it just tell me everything all at once?"

Andreas smiled, understanding his frustration. "If you asked a human expert to tell you everything they know about cancer, they'd be overwhelmed. Their knowledge is vast, but it's stored in a way that requires specific questions to access. Cancerase GPT works the same way. It has a vast amount of knowledge, but it's stored in a neural network that requires prompts to bring it to the surface. You're guiding the conversation, shaping the responses by what you ask."

Dr. Dean stared at the computer screen, his frustration slowly giving way to curiosity. "So, if I wanted to write a scientific article on the use of herbal medicine in cancer treatment, I'd have to start by asking specific questions about each herb and its effects?"

"Exactly," Andreas said encouragingly. "You could start by asking Cancerase GPT about the effectiveness of certain herbs, the latest research, or even case studies. Then, based on its answers, you refine your questions to go deeper into the topics that interest you."

Dr. Dean nodded slowly. "Okay, I think I'm starting to understand. It's not just about getting information; it's about having a dialogue, just like I would with a colleague or a patient."

Andreas grinned. "Now you've got it! Cancerase GPT is an invaluable tool, but it's the human element—our ability to ask the right questions and guide the narrative—that truly brings an article to life. Writing with Cancerase GPT isn't about pushing a button; it's about pulling knowledge out, piece by piece, just like you would from any expert."

Dr. Dean smiled for the first time that afternoon. "Alright, let's give this another try. Cancerase GPT, tell me about the latest advancements in herbal medicine for breast cancer. And don't hold back—give me everything you've got!"

The computer screen flickered, and the AI began to generate a detailed response, full of insights and information. Dr. Dean leaned in, his frustration forgotten, replaced by a newfound sense of excitement and curiosity. He was starting to see the potential of this strange, digital assistant—and maybe, just maybe, he was beginning to understand how to work with it.

Andreas watched with a satisfied smile as Dr. Dean began to engage with Cancerase GPT, asking more specific questions and getting deeper into the topic. It wasn't exactly like pressing a magic button, but it was something even better: a true collaboration between human and machine, each bringing their unique strengths to the table.

Dr. Dean looked up from the screen, a twinkle in his eye. "You know, Andreas, this might just work after all. I think we're going to write one heck of a scientific article." Andreas laughed. "That's the spirit, Dr. Dean. Now let's see what else Cancerase GPT can do!"

With that, they continued their journey, exploring the depths of Cancerase GPT's knowledge, one prompt at a time, and discovering that sometimes, the most powerful tool in writing isn't a button—it's a question.

Chapter 13: The Forgotten Miracle Drugs

"The most powerful remedies are often hidden in plain sight, buried beneath the weight of profit-driven priorities. Medicine should be a pursuit of healing, not just a business of innovation. Sometimes, the real breakthroughs are not the newest or the most expensive—they are the forgotten, the overlooked, and the unprofitable. True progress lies in the courage to rediscover what has always worked and the wisdom to use it for the greater good."
Andreas Kazmierczak

The IV room had become a classroom of sorts for Andreas and Dr. Dean. With Andreas having explained the complexities of AI and machine learning, it was now Dr. Dean's turn to share his wealth of knowledge on integrative cancer treatment. Dr. Dean, a seasoned expert in holistic health, was eager to teach Andreas, but little did he know that his AI engineer friend had a knack for taking things quite literally.

"All right, Andreas," Dr. Dean began, setting aside his papers, "today I'm going to teach you about the integrative methods we use in cancer treatment—off-label drugs, antibiotics, repurposed medications, the whole spectrum. These treatments work together to support the body's natural healing processes and disrupt cancer's ability to spread."

Andreas nodded enthusiastically. "I'm ready, Dr. Dean! Hit me with the knowledge!"

Dr. Dean chuckled. "Let's start with something simple. Have you ever heard of Tagamet?"

"The heartburn medication?" Andreas asked, raising an eyebrow. "What, do cancer cells get indigestion?"

Dr. Dean laughed. "Not exactly. Tagamet, or cimetidine, is an H2 blocker typically used to treat acid reflux. But here's the interesting part—studies have shown that it can help inhibit cancer metastasis, particularly in gastrointestinal and colorectal cancers. It works by blocking histamine receptors, which are involved in cancer cell growth and immune suppression."

Andreas tilted his head. "So… we're giving cancer a bad case of acid reflux to slow it down?"

Dr. Dean smirked. "If that helps you remember it, sure. But the real magic is how it enhances the immune system's ability to fight cancer by reducing T-regulatory cells, which otherwise suppress the body's natural defenses against tumors. It has been particularly useful post-surgery to prevent circulating tumor cells (CTCs) from settling in new locations."

Andreas' eyes lit up. "That sounds like a firewall for cancer. I like it. What else you got?"

Dr. Dean leaned in. "Now let's talk about something even more interesting—Doxycycline."

Andreas furrowed his brow. "Wait, isn't that just an antibiotic? What does it have to do with cancer?"

Dr. Dean grinned. "A lot more than you'd think. Doxycycline isn't just for infections—it's a mitochondrial disruptor. Cancer stem cells rely on their mitochondria for survival and energy production, and doxycycline messes with that process. It targets circulating tumor cells (CTCs) and cancer stem cells (CSCs) by cutting off their energy supply, making them more vulnerable to other therapies."

Andreas whistled. "So, we're basically hacking the cancer's

power source? That's genius."

"Exactly," Dr. Dean nodded. "And when you combine it with something like Vitamin C or metronomic chemotherapy, it weakens the cancer cells even more, making them easier to destroy."

Andreas tapped his chin. "I see where this is going. So, if we're shutting down the cancer's fuel, what's next? Do we send in a cleanup crew?"

Dr. Dean grinned. "That's where Niclosamide comes in."

"The deworming drug? You're telling me we're treating cancer like a parasite?"

Dr. Dean chuckled. "In a way, yes. Niclosamide has been used for decades to treat tapeworm infections, but it also has some impressive anti-cancer properties. It disrupts cancer cell signaling pathways, like Wnt/β-catenin, which is crucial for cancer cell survival and metastasis."

Andreas leaned forward, fascinated. "So, it's like cutting the cancer's internet connection?"

"Precisely," Dr. Dean said. "Niclosamide prevents cancer cells from communicating and coordinating their survival tactics. On top of that, it also reduces inflammation, suppresses drug resistance mechanisms, and targets cancer stem cells, making it an incredible addition to an integrative cancer treatment plan."

Andreas shook his head, grinning. "So, we're treating cancer with heartburn meds, antibiotics, and a deworming pill? This sounds like the weirdest medicine cabinet ever."

Dr. Dean laughed. "That's the beauty of repurposed drugs. We're using safe, already-approved medications in new and innovative ways to fight cancer more effectively. And the best part? These drugs are cheap, widely available, and come with decades of safety data."

Andreas leaned back, impressed. "It's like open-source medicine. Instead of waiting decades for new drugs, we're reusing existing ones in smarter ways."

"Exactly," Dr. Dean said, smiling. "And the more we refine our AI with this knowledge, the better we can tailor treatments for each patient. Cancerase AI could become a global database for the best combinations, making personalized treatment accessible to everyone."

Andreas nodded, feeling a new wave of inspiration. "You know, Dr. Dean, this is starting to sound less like medicine and more like a battle strategy. We're hitting cancer from all angles— cutting off its supply lines, disrupting its communication, and attacking its defenses all at once."

Dr. Dean grinned. "That's exactly what we're doing, Andreas. And with AI on our side, we're just getting started."

As the two continued their discussion, Andreas realized that this wasn't just about medicine—it was about changing the way cancer was fought forever. With a mix of science, strategy, and a touch of creativity, they were crafting a new frontier in integrative oncology, one breakthrough at a time.

Chapter 14: The Parasitic Nature of Cancer

"What if cancer is not just a mutation, but an invader? Like a parasite, it hijacks, consumes, and spreads without regard for its host. And if we treat it as such, using the same strategies that have defeated parasites for centuries, we might uncover a new way to fight back. The greatest breakthroughs often come not from new discoveries, but from re-examining what we thought we already knew." Andreas Kazmierczak

In the dim glow of the IV room, with the soft beeping of machines filling the space, Dr. Dean leaned forward, his expression intense. Andreas had seen him serious before, but this was different—there was something almost urgent in his demeanor.

"Andreas," Dr. Dean began, folding his hands together, "there's something about cancer that modern medicine has largely overlooked or perhaps chosen to ignore. I want to talk to you about a radical, yet increasingly validated idea—cancer as a parasitic disease."

Andreas frowned, clearly intrigued but skeptical. "A parasitic disease? I thought cancer was just mutated cells growing uncontrollably?"

Dr. Dean nodded. "That's the mainstream understanding, yes. But let's look deeper. Cancer behaves in ways eerily similar to parasites. It hijacks the body's resources, evades the immune system, spreads aggressively, and—most paradoxically—kills its host. Tell me, Andreas, why would a disease evolve to kill its own host when survival should be its primary goal?"

Andreas rubbed his chin, considering the point. "You're right. That doesn't make much sense from an evolutionary standpoint.

Most biological organisms fight to survive, not destroy their environment."

"Exactly!" Dr. Dean's eyes gleamed. "Look at parasitic infections—malaria, certain bacterial infections, and even fungi like candida. They invade, they feed, they spread, and they often kill their hosts.

This goes against the fundamental instinct of life. Why would cancer do the same? What if—just what if—cancer isn't just a genetic mutation but something far more sinister?"

Andreas sat back, exhaling slowly. "Are you saying cancer is...a parasite?"

"Not in the traditional sense, no," Dr. Dean admitted. "But it behaves in a way that mimics parasitic infections. And here's where things get interesting. Some oncologists have been experimenting with anti-parasitic drugs like Ivermectin, Mebendazole, and Hydroxychloroquine—and they're seeing results."

Andreas's eyebrows shot up. "Wait. You mean these drugs, originally designed for parasites, are actually killing cancer?"

Dr. Dean nodded. "Yes, and not just killing it—outperforming chemotherapy in some cases. There's an oncologist in Japan who has been testing Mebendazole and Hydroxychloroquine together, and the results have been astounding.

The combination is proving more effective than conventional chemotherapy. These drugs disrupt the cancer's ability to grow, spread, and even protect itself from the immune system."

Andreas was silent for a long moment, absorbing this revelation.

"But why isn't this common knowledge? If these treatments work, why aren't they being used worldwide?"

Dr. Dean sighed. "That's the problem, Andreas. Cancer treatment is a multi-billion-dollar industry. Chemotherapy, radiation, and targeted therapies dominate the market. Off-patent drugs like Mebendazole and Ivermectin don't generate the same kind of profit. There's little financial incentive for large pharmaceutical companies to fund studies on these alternatives."

Andreas clenched his jaw. "That's insane. If these medications are working, then we need to push this information out there."

Dr. Dean leaned back. "That's exactly why we're doing this with Cancerase GPT. The medical world needs more than just AI-powered knowledge—it needs access to suppressed truths, alternative perspectives, and the best possible treatment options for patients, regardless of profit margins."

Andreas exhaled sharply. "This changes everything. It's almost as if cancer is more than just a disease—it's something unnatural, something...evil."

Dr. Dean nodded solemnly. "And that's why it requires an unconventional approach. If we treat it like a parasite, using anti-parasitic drugs, we might be able to fight it more effectively than we ever thought possible."

The two men sat in silence for a moment, the weight of their discussion settling between them. Andreas finally spoke. "Then we have work to do. We need to dive deeper, find more evidence, and make sure this information reaches the people who need it."

Dr. Dean smiled. "That's exactly what I was hoping you'd say."

The hum of the machines around them felt different now—less like background noise and more like the pulse of something new, something revolutionary. Together, they were on the verge of redefining cancer treatment, and perhaps, unlocking one of medicine's greatest mysteries.

Chapter 15: The Complexity of Cancer – An Engineer's Perspective

"Cancer is not a single enemy but a complex battlefield of evolving variables. A one-size-fits-all approach is like navigating the cosmos with a compass. AI isn't a replacement for human expertise but an ally—capable of processing vast data, recognizing hidden patterns, and crafting treatment strategies as unique as each patient. The future of cancer care is intelligence-driven."

Andreas Kazmierczak

The soft hum of machines and the faint scent of antiseptics lingered in the IV room as Andreas leaned forward, his hands gesturing with the precision of an engineer deep in thought. Across from him sat Dr. Dean, an experienced oncologist with decades of medical knowledge, but someone who had never quite seen cancer through the lens that Andreas was about to introduce.

"Dr. Dean," Andreas began, his voice measured yet passionate, "I come from a world where complexity isn't just expected—it's the very foundation of our work. As an engineer, I spend my days solving intricate problems that require multi-layered solutions. There's never a single answer, never a magic button that instantly fixes everything. And yet, when I look at modern oncology, I see an approach that attempts to reduce cancer—one of the most complex biological phenomena—to a singular solution."

Dr. Dean raised an eyebrow, intrigued. "What do you mean by that?"

Andreas leaned back, choosing his words carefully. "Imagine someone tells you that flying to the moon is simple—just build a rocket and launch it. But you and I both know that's absurd.

A moon landing requires an enormous amount of planning, calculations, engineering, and problem-solving. Every single component has to work in harmony. You need propulsion, life support, navigation, fuel efficiency, aerodynamics, and so much more. It's an incredibly complex system with thousands of variables."

Dr. Dean nodded slowly. "And you're saying cancer is just as complex?"

"Even more so," Andreas replied firmly. "Cancer isn't just one disease; it's a collection of thousands of diseases, all with different causes, behaviors, and responses to treatment. And yet, modern medicine often tries to simplify it—radiation will heal everything, or chemotherapy will make the cancer disappear. That's like saying one single design can launch every spacecraft in existence. It doesn't work that way. Each case of cancer is unique and needs a tailored, multi-faceted approach."

Dr. Dean folded his arms, considering this perspective. "So, in your view, what's missing in oncology?"

Andreas exhaled, tapping his fingers on the table. "The first thing that's missing is a deeper understanding of the source of cancer. In engineering, we never try to solve a problem without first diagnosing it properly. But in medicine, we often attack cancer without truly understanding what caused it in the first place. Was it genetic? Environmental? Metabolic? Viral? A combination? Until we identify the root cause, how can we possibly develop the right treatment?"

Dr. Dean sighed. "That's a fair point. Medicine tends to treat the symptoms, not always the origin."

"Exactly," Andreas agreed. "And the second thing missing is the right tool to handle this level of complexity. Human doctors, no matter how brilliant, simply cannot process millions of data points, analyze intricate biochemical pathways, and predict the best course of treatment for each individual patient. But AI can."

Dr. Dean frowned slightly. "You believe AI can do what humans cannot?"

Andreas nodded. "Think about it—AI has the capacity to analyze vast amounts of medical literature, patient histories, genetic information, and treatment responses all at once. It doesn't get tired, it doesn't have biases, and it can identify patterns that we would never see. AI can take into account the patient's unique cancer type, their biomarkers, their immune system response, their diet, lifestyle, and even psychological factors. Then, it can generate a personalized treatment plan that incorporates a combination of medications, natural compounds, dietary changes, and alternative methods—whatever has the highest likelihood of success."

Dr. Dean sat in silence for a moment, absorbing Andreas's words. "That's a radical shift from traditional oncology," he admitted. "Most doctors are trained to rely on standardized protocols."

"And that's the problem," Andreas replied. "Standardized protocols assume that all cancers are the same, but they're not. Cancer is not an infection. With infections, we know the exact cause—a bacteria, a virus, a fungus. We understand how the body reacts, and we have antibiotics and antiviral drugs that directly target these pathogens. But cancer? Cancer is a biological enigma. To believe there is one universal 'cancer cure' is naive. It will never be that simple."

Dr. Dean exhaled sharply. "So, what you're proposing is a

shift from a one-size-fits-all model to an AI-driven, hyper-personalized approach to cancer treatment."

Andreas smiled. "Exactly. AI is the only tool we have that can handle this level of complexity. It can continuously learn, refine its models, and optimize treatments for each individual. It's the bridge between the chaos of cancer and the precision we need to fight it effectively."

Dr. Dean nodded slowly. "I have to admit, Andreas, I've never quite thought about cancer this way. You're right—it's not a single problem with a single solution. It's a vast, interconnected system of challenges that require an equally intricate approach. And AI... AI might just be the missing piece."

A sense of understanding passed between them, an acknowledgment that a new frontier in cancer treatment was emerging. As they sat in the quiet hum of the IV room, it became clear that medicine was on the cusp of a revolution— one where engineering, data science, and artificial intelligence would illuminate the path to better, smarter, and more effective cancer treatments.

Andreas leaned forward, his eyes full of determination. "We're standing at the threshold of something huge, Dr. Dean. And I think we both know—it's time to step through."

Chapter 16: A Dinner to Remember - The Birth of LYFBLEND

"The most powerful ideas are born at the crossroads of tradition and innovation. When wisdom of the past meets the technology of the future, we create solutions that not only heal—but redefine the way we live." Andreas Kazmierczak

It was a warm evening as Andreas and his wife, Isabell, walked into the cozy little Florida restaurant where they were meeting Dr. Dean and his fiancée, April. The four had become close over the past few months, united not only by their shared battle against cancer but also by their common mission to change the world of cancer treatment. Tonight was a celebration—a chance to relax, enjoy good food, and discuss the exciting progress of Cancerase GPT.

As they sat down, Isabell looked at Andreas, a mischievous smile playing on her lips. "So, how's everything going with Cancerase GPT? Any breakthroughs since the last dinner?"

Andreas grinned. "You know me, I never stop working. The AI's getting smarter every day. It's actually starting to surprise me."

April, ever the optimist, leaned forward. "Smart AI and big dreams, I like it. But I'm curious—what's next? We've talked a lot about Cancerase GPT helping patients, but is there something more tangible we can offer? Something people can actually take home?"

Dr. Dean, who had been listening intently, nodded. "Funny you mention that, April. I've been thinking along those lines myself. We've got this treasure trove of knowledge from both my personal experience and Cancerase GPT's capabilities. What if we could create something physical? A supplement that could help support cancer prevention or assist with treatment?"

Isabell raised an eyebrow, intrigued. "A supplement, huh? You're really going to convince me to swallow something every day, Dr. Dean?"

"Not just any supplement," Dr. Dean clarified. "I'm thinking a nutraceutical blend, something that combines the best of natural medicine and the latest scientific findings from Cancerase GPT. We'd blend traditional herbs with cutting-edge data."

April's eyes lit up. "So, you're telling me this is going to be the magic pill? A combination of ancient wisdom and modern science?"

Andreas chuckled. "Magic pill? I think April's already thinking about how to market it."

April shrugged playfully. "I'm just saying—if we're going to change cancer treatment, we might as well make it sound like we're doing something revolutionary."

Isabell, always the voice of reason, leaned in. "But seriously, how would we decide what goes into this blend? Are we just picking ingredients that sound good or is there an actual strategy?"

"That's where Cancerase GPT comes in," Dr. Dean explained. "We'll use it to analyze all the research—both scientific studies and traditional knowledge—about the most effective herbs and nutrients. The AI will help us determine what works best for cancer prevention and treatment. We'll make sure it's a scientifically backed, perfectly balanced formula."

April clapped her hands together. "I love it. This is exactly what we need! We could call it **LYFBLEND**. A blend of life—vibrant health, longevity, and cancer prevention."

Isabell laughed. "LYFBLEND, huh? I can already picture the marketing campaign. It's catchy!"

Andreas grinned. "And it sounds like something you could drink while lounging on a beach. I'm sold."

The group continued to brainstorm over their meal, discussing potential ingredients for LYFBLEND. Dr. Dean, with his wealth of knowledge about integrative medicine, suggested turmeric for its anti-inflammatory and anti-cancer properties, and green tea extract for its potent antioxidants. April, always thinking about natural healing, added ideas like ginger to reduce nausea and boost immunity, and milk thistle for liver detoxification.

Isabell looked thoughtful. "But we need something to tie it all together. Something that makes this more than just a supplement—it needs to be something that will resonate with people."

April nodded. "Exactly. And what better way to tie it all together than by using the power of AI to create something that evolves over time? We could adjust the formula as new research comes out, always staying on the cutting edge."

Andreas leaned back in his chair, already brainstorming the technical side of things. "We could have Cancerase GPT continually analyze new studies, running simulations to ensure that every new iteration of LYFBLEND is optimized. It could even adjust the ratios of ingredients based on the latest cancer research. The possibilities are endless."

Dr. Dean raised his glass. "So, we're agreed then. We'll use the AI to create a blend that's rooted in science and nature, and LYFBLEND will be our first step in changing the cancer treatment landscape."

April clinked her glass with his. "To LYFBLEND, to science, and to the most unpredictable, health-conscious team I've ever been part of."

Isabell smiled, shaking her head. "I never thought I'd be in a restaurant brainstorming cancer treatment while talking about turmeric and ginger."

Andreas laughed. "I never thought I'd be sitting at dinner wondering if I need a supplement to improve my AI's cognitive function."

The group clinked their glasses together again, united in their shared mission. They weren't just creating a product—they were creating a movement, one that would bring together the wisdom of the past and the technology of the future to offer something truly revolutionary. And with LYFBLEND, they were ready to take the next step.

As they left the restaurant that evening, the group felt a renewed sense of purpose. They were not just friends or colleagues—they were pioneers, ready to change the world of cancer treatment, one blend at a time.

Chapter 17: The Power of Metabolic Therapy

"Cancer thrives in the shadows of metabolic dysfunction. By shifting the body's energy sources, enhancing mitochondrial function, and depriving cancer of its fuel, we turn its greatest strength into its weakness. The key to treatment is not just in killing cancer—but in outsmarting it." Andreas Kazmierczak

Andreas sat across from Dr. Dean, his mind still processing the discussions they had over the past few weeks. They had explored alternative therapies, repurposed drugs, and integrative treatments—but one concept kept resurfacing: metabolism.

"Dr. Dean," Andreas started, rubbing his chin. "We've talked about starving cancer with glucose restriction, but what about shifting the body's metabolism entirely? Can we rewire it to fight cancer from the inside?"

Dr. Dean nodded. "That's exactly what metabolic therapy is about. Instead of only targeting cancer cells with external treatments, we change the body's entire biochemical environment to make it inhospitable to cancer growth."

Andreas leaned forward, intrigued. "How does that work?"

Dr. Dean grabbed a notepad and began sketching a rough diagram of a cell. "Cancer cells rely heavily on glycolysis for energy, even in the presence of oxygen. It's called the Warburg effect. Unlike healthy cells, which use the mitochondria to generate energy efficiently, cancer cells prefer to ferment glucose. It's an inefficient process, but it allows them to survive in low-oxygen environments. So, what if we cut off that pathway and force them to rely on their damaged mitochondria?"

Andreas' eyes lit up. "That would be a death sentence for them, wouldn't it?"

"Exactly," Dr. Dean said with a smile. "One of the most promising strategies is the ketogenic diet—eliminating sugar and carbohydrates while increasing healthy fats and ketones. When the body switches from glucose metabolism to ketone metabolism, cancer cells struggle to adapt. They don't have the metabolic flexibility of normal cells."

Andreas exhaled, his engineering mind racing with the implications. "So, by shifting the fuel source, we're essentially taking away cancer's main advantage?"

Dr. Dean nodded. "But it doesn't stop there. There are compounds that can enhance this metabolic shift even further— things like hyperbaric oxygen therapy, which increases oxygen saturation and forces cancer cells into oxidative stress. There's also dichloroacetate (DCA), which helps restore mitochondrial function in cancer cells, pushing them toward apoptosis instead of uncontrolled growth."

Andreas tapped his fingers on the table. "And all of this… it's not mainstream treatment?"

Dr. Dean sighed. "No, because it doesn't involve a billion-dollar drug. The pharmaceutical industry focuses on targeted therapies that attack specific mutations, but they overlook the bigger picture. Cancer isn't just a genetic disease—it's a metabolic one. If we treat it at the metabolic level, we don't need to chase every mutation individually. We disrupt the entire system that cancer relies on."

Andreas shook his head in disbelief. "So, with the right diet, metabolic therapies, and a strategic use of supplements, we could weaken cancer before it even has a chance to grow?"

"Exactly," Dr. Dean said. "Think of it like structural engineering. If you wanted to destroy a bridge, you wouldn't just chip away at individual bricks. You'd weaken the foundation, cut off the supply lines, and let gravity do the rest. That's what we're doing with metabolic therapy—we're attacking cancer at its foundation."

Andreas sat back, feeling a mix of frustration and excitement. "So why isn't this part of every cancer treatment plan?"

Dr. Dean chuckled. "Because medicine moves slowly, and profits move quickly. But that's why we're here—to change the conversation. With AI-driven analysis, we can compile the research, identify the best metabolic strategies, and create personalized protocols that give patients the best chance at survival."

Andreas nodded, a determined glint in his eyes. "Then let's make it happen. If we can teach people how to fight cancer at the metabolic level, we're not just treating the disease—we're changing the game entirely."

As the IV machine continued its steady rhythm, Andreas knew they were onto something far greater than a single treatment. They were redefining the way cancer was understood, treated, and ultimately defeated.

Chapter 18: The Future of Cancer Treatment

"The future of cancer treatment lies not in one-size-fits-all solutions, but in precision, collaboration, and intelligence. By integrating genomic data, real-time monitoring, and AI-driven insights, we move beyond treating cancer to truly understanding it. The revolution begins when medicine, technology, and human ingenuity unite—not just to fight cancer, but to outsmart it." Andreas Kazmierczak

As the sun dipped below the horizon, casting a warm glow over the clinic, Andreas and Dr. Dean sat together in the IV room. The hum of machines and the soft beeping of monitors filled the space, but their conversation had shifted from treatment to something greater—the future.

"Dr. Dean," Andreas began, his voice firm yet thoughtful, "we both know that cancer is far too complex for a single doctor to handle alone. The way we've been treating cancer—relying on one-size-fits-all solutions—is fundamentally flawed. The only way forward is through large, interdisciplinary teams that bring together the brightest minds from medicine, and artificial intelligence."

Dr. Dean nodded. "I couldn't agree more. The traditional approach—where a doctor prescribes chemotherapy or radiation as a singular cure—is outdated. Cancer isn't a single disease; it's a collection of thousands of unique conditions, each with its own triggers, mutations, and weaknesses. The future of oncology must be individualized, precise, and based on deep, scientific understanding."

Andreas leaned forward. "Exactly. Personalized genomic testing is already revolutionizing cancer treatment. In Germany, one of the global leaders in cancer research, patients can now undergo tests that measure the exact amount of circulating tumor cells in their bloodstream. These tests don't just confirm the presence of cancer—they identify the most effective chemotherapy agents for each patient, optimizing treatment and minimizing side effects."

Dr. Dean smiled. "And it doesn't stop there. Switzerland is pioneering another critical approach—testing cancer cells against a variety of treatments to determine their specific vulnerabilities. With this data, oncologists can craft personalized treatment plans that not only attack the cancer effectively but also prevent recurrence. The era of blindly prescribing toxic drugs is ending. Science is finally catching up with the complexity of this disease."

Andreas exhaled. "And yet, despite these advancements, mainstream medicine is still slow to adopt them. Cancer treatment is too often dictated by financial incentives rather than scientific progress. Pharmaceutical companies prioritize expensive, long-term therapies over cost-effective solutions. We have to take financial motives out of the equation. Only then can we truly revolutionize cancer care."

Dr. Dean nodded solemnly. "The industry's focus on profitability has indeed hindered progress. But we are at a turning point. Oxygen therapy, thermal therapy, cryotherapy—these methods have shown great promise against cancer, yet they remain underutilized because they don't generate the same profit as patented drugs. We need to integrate these methods into standard treatment protocols."

Andreas saw the parallels between medicine and engineering clearly. "You know, Dr. Dean, in engineering, when we build complex structures—bridges, spacecraft, or AI systems—we start with data. We test materials, analyze environmental conditions, and run simulations. We don't assume that one material or one method will work universally. Cancer treatment should follow the same principles. Every patient is different. We need extensive data collection, real-time monitoring, and AI-driven analysis to construct the best possible treatment plans."

Dr. Dean smiled. "That's exactly why Cancerase GPT is so important. AI has the potential to process millions of data points in ways no human ever could. It can cross-reference genomic profiles, past case studies, and emerging treatments to generate highly personalized protocols. The future of oncology isn't just about doctors—it's about teams of experts and intelligent AI systems working together."

Andreas felt a surge of determination. "Then that's our mission. To change the narrative, to build an approach that isn't just reactive but predictive. Cancer shouldn't just be treated—it should be understood at its root cause, and then eradicated with precision."

Dr. Dean extended his hand, and Andreas clasped it firmly. "We've only scratched the surface, Andreas. The real revolution in cancer treatment is just beginning."

As they sat in the quiet hum of the clinic, the weight of their discussion settled between them. This wasn't just about medicine—it was about the future of human health, about reshaping the way the world confronted one of its deadliest diseases. And in that moment, both men knew they were part of something much larger than themselves.

A new era in cancer treatment was dawning.

Epilogue: Embracing Hope and the Future of Cancer Care

"The future of cancer care lies not in a single cure but in the synergy of knowledge, technology, and the human spirit. When we integrate the wisdom of traditional medicine, the precision of science, and the power of AI, we transform cancer from an inevitable fate into a challenge that can be overcome. Hope is not just a feeling—it is the bridge between innovation and healing, leading us to a world where every patient has the tools to fight, the knowledge to choose, and the support to thrive." <small>Andreas Kazmierczak</small>

As we reach the end of this journey through the many facets of integrative cancer care, we want to leave you with a message of hope. This book has explored a wide range of treatments, therapies, and strategies that span the globe, from ancient practices to cutting-edge technologies. And yet, this is only the beginning. We stand on the brink of a new era in medicine, one where cancer does not have to be a life sentence but a challenge that can be met with resilience, innovation, and a holistic approach to healing.

For Patients: Your Journey of Hope

If you are reading this chapter, you or someone you love is likely facing the daunting challenge of cancer. It's a journey filled with uncertainty, fear, and moments of deep despair. But it is also a journey filled with opportunity—an opportunity to explore new treatments, discover hidden strengths within yourself, and transform your life in ways you never thought possible.

Remember, cancer is not just a disease of the body; it affects your mind, spirit, and every aspect of your life. That's why integrative cancer care is so powerful. It recognizes you as a whole person and aims to support your body's natural ability to heal while also addressing the emotional, psychological, and spiritual dimensions of your journey.

Throughout this book, we have shared the stories of those who have walked this path before you, individuals who have faced the same fears and challenges but found hope and healing through integrative methods. Their stories, like yours, are powerful testaments to the resilience of the human spirit and the potential for recovery, even in the face of the most daunting odds.

While no two journeys are the same, there is a common thread that binds all those who face cancer: the desire to live fully, to love deeply, and to find meaning in each day. This is your story, and you have the power to shape it in ways that reflect your deepest values and highest hopes. Never forget that you are not alone. A community of fellow travelers, dedicated doctors, and caring professionals stand ready to support you every step of the way.

For Doctors: Embracing New Methods and Integrating AI

To our fellow healthcare professionals, we extend a call to action. The field of cancer care is evolving rapidly, and the integration of new methods and technologies is not just an option but a necessity. We are living in a time of unprecedented scientific discovery, where integrative therapies, precision medicine, and AI-driven insights offer new hope to our patients.

As doctors, we have the privilege and the responsibility to explore all possible avenues to help those in our care. We must be open to learning from global traditions, incorporating evidence-based complementary therapies, and embracing the technological advancements that AI brings to the table. This book has outlined various integrative approaches that have shown promise in supporting conventional cancer treatments, enhancing patient well-being, and, in some cases, achieving remarkable outcomes.

AI is rapidly changing the landscape of medicine. It has the potential to revolutionize how we understand cancer at the molecular level, predict how it behaves, and personalize treatments like never before. AI algorithms can analyze vast amounts of data, identifying patterns and correlations that humans alone could not detect. This could lead to breakthroughs in how we approach prevention, diagnosis, and treatment—possibly even finding a cure.

Imagine a world where AI can predict the best treatment plan for each individual, where nutrition and lifestyle modifications are tailored precisely to the genetic makeup and cancer profile of every patient. Imagine an AI system that continuously learns from every patient's experience, refining its recommendations to increase effectiveness and reduce side effects. This is not science fiction; it is a future that is being built right now.

Looking Forward: A Future Filled with Possibility

The fight against cancer is far from over, but we are not fighting it in the same way we did a decade ago, or even a few years ago. The integration of new knowledge, diverse healing practices, and cutting-edge technology gives us more tools and greater hope than ever before.

We envision a future where cancer care is not limited to the walls of a hospital or the confines of a single treatment protocol. It will be a dynamic, evolving field where patients are empowered with knowledge, doctors are armed with the latest tools, and AI plays a crucial role in delivering personalized, precise care.

This future is not just about prolonging life but enhancing its quality. It is about ensuring that every person diagnosed with cancer has access to the most advanced treatments available, the support to navigate their journey with dignity, and the hope that comes from knowing they are not alone.

As we close this chapter, we urge you to keep moving forward with courage and hope. For patients, continue to seek knowledge, ask questions, and embrace the full spectrum of care available to you. For doctors, continue to push the boundaries of what is possible, stay curious, and remain open to the new tools and methods that can help us in our shared mission to conquer cancer.

Together, we can create a future where cancer is not a word that instills fear but a challenge that can be met with strength, knowledge, and the unwavering support of a community dedicated to healing.

Let this be the start of a new chapter in your life—a chapter filled with hope, resilience, and the endless possibilities that the future of cancer care holds.

23. Bibliography

The bibliography for this book is not presented in a static, printed form. Instead, readers can find the most up-to-date references and sources on our dedicated website:

https://cangpt.ai

The reason for this dynamic approach is that the artificial intelligence (AI) system that verified the data in this book is constantly evolving. Each day, it learns new facts, clinical outcomes, and advancements in integrative cancer treatments. The field of oncology is progressing at a rapid pace, and we believe that a fixed bibliography would quickly become outdated.

By hosting the bibliography online, we ensure that readers have access to the latest scientific research, innovative therapies, emerging products, and novel ideas. The book itself is updated almost every month, reflecting the newest insights from **CANCERASE GPT AI (https://cangpt.ai)**, an ever-expanding repository of knowledge designed to stay at the forefront of integrative cancer care.

We encourage readers to visit the website regularly, not only to check the most current sources but also to download the latest version of the book. As the AI grows smarter and smarter with each passing month, we are committed to sharing that growth and the valuable information it uncovers with you, our readers.

23.1. Example of How to Use the Bibliography

This book introduces a new genre of bibliography. All the information you will find in this book is based on a knowledge AI system, trained by the experienced oncologist Dr. Dean Silver. Every thesis or data presented in the book includes a reference to the page number and the source name within the AI system. The AI system lists all the materials it was trained on through the website cangpt.ai.

For example, the book provides a reference for a particular thesis, such as "document-3456, page 1." On the website cangpt.ai, you can find a table with the document number and a link to the page where the document is hosted.

23.2. Important Things to Know About the Book

The book itself is updated almost every month, reflecting the newest insights from CANCERASE GPT AI, an ever-expanding repository of knowledge designed to stay at the forefront of integrative cancer care.

We encourage readers to visit the website regularly, not only to check the most current sources but also to download the latest version of the book. As the AI grows smarter and smarter with each passing month, we are committed to sharing that growth and the valuable information it uncovers with you, our readers.

Index

104

patient histories 86

patients 8, 12–13, 16, 18, 21, 25–27, 31, 35, 41, 44–46, 55–56, 58–59, 82, 88, 94, 96, 98–101

patterns 11, 28, 31, 63, 84, 86, 100

pelvic radiation 54

personalized medicine 14

personalized treatment 12, 79, 86, 96

personalized treatment plans 96

PET scans 44

pharmaceutical commissions 58

pharmaceutical companies 40, 82, 96

pharmaceutical industry 58, 93

phytonutrients 35

Pinecone 24, 29

Pini viscum 67

plant-based 15–16, 35, 43

precision medicine 7, 99

precision-driven 14

predictions 28

pro-oxidant 48, 53, 55

probability 63, 65

processed food 34

programming language 30

prompts 72, 74

prostate 52, 63–64

prostate cancer 52, 63

protocol 57, 100

Python 23, 30

Q

R

radiation 7, 11, 16, 53–54, 63–64, 82, 85, 95

radiation therapy 54

radical prostatectomy 52

radiologist 53

recommendations 25, 100

recurrence 16, 53–54, 63–65, 96

remission 18–19, 24, 52

repurposed drugs 15–17, 38, 78, 92

repurposed medications 76

research 8, 12–13, 15, 19–21, 25, 30–31, 45, 53, 74, 89–90, 94, 96, 102, 658

research assistant 30

responses 29, 31, 74, 85–86

resveratrol 45

revolution in cancer care 45

RNA 41

S

sales tactics 57

science 11, 14–17, 20, 26, 43–44, 58, 79, 87, 89–91, 96, 98, 100

scientific article 72–75

scientific articles 24, 30

scientific studies and traditional knowledge 89

selenium 16

side effects 40–41, 45–46, 48–50, 54, 96, 100

spice 34–35, 37

standardized protocols 86

statistics 9, 63–65

success rates 65

sugar 39, 41, 93

suggestions 20

super-fast 30

supplements 25, 41, 55, 57, 60, 62, 93

suppressed truths 11, 82

www.ingramcontent.com/pod-product-compliance
Lightning Source LLC
Chambersburg PA
CBHW031215270326
41931CB00006B/573